Complications in Facial Plastic Surgery

Editors

RICHARD L. GOODE
SAM P. MOST

FACIAL PLASTIC SURGERY CLINICS OF NORTH AMERICA

www.facialplastic.theclinics.com

Consulting Editor
J. REGAN THOMAS

November 2013 • Volume 21 • Number 4

ELSEVIER

1600 John F. Kennedy Boulevard • Suite 1800 • Philadelphia, Pennsylvania, 19103-2899

http://www.theclinics.com

FACIAL PLASTIC SURGERY CLINICS OF NORTH AMERICA Volume 21, Number 4
November 2013 ISSN 1064-7406, ISBN-13: 978-0-323-24221-9

Editor: Joanne Husovski
Developmental Editor: Susan Showalter

Facial Plastic Surgery Clinics of North America (ISSN 1064-7406) is published quarterly by Elsevier Inc., 360 Park Avenue South, New York, NY 10010-1710. Months of issue are February, May, August, and November. Business and Editorial Offices: 1600 John F. Kennedy Blvd., Suite 1800, Philadelphia, PA 19103-2899. Periodicals postage paid at New York, NY, and additional mailing offices. Subscription prices are $373.00 per year (US individuals), $526.00 per year (US institutions), $425.00 per year (Canadian individuals), $628.00 per year (Canadian institutions), $509.00 per year (foreign individuals), $628.00 per year (foreign institutions), $153.00 per year (US students), and $245.00 per year (foreign students). Foreign air speed delivery is included in all *Clinics* subscription prices. All prices are subject to change without notice. POSTMASTER: Send address changes to *Facial Plastic Surgery Clinics*, Elsevier Health Sciences Division, Subscription Customer Service, 3251 Riverport Lane, Maryland Heights, MO 63043. **Customer service: 1-800-654-2452 (US and Canada); 1-314-447-8871 (outside US and Canada); Fax: 314-447-8029; E-mail:journalscustomerservice-usa@elsevier.com (for print support); journalsonline support-usa@elsevier.com (for online support).**

Reprints. For copies of 100 or more of articles in this publication, please contact the Commercial Reprints Department, Elsevier Inc., 360 Park Avenue South, New York, NY 10010-1710. Tel.: 212-633-3874; Fax: 212-633-3820; E-mail: reprints@elsevier.com.

Facial Plastic Surgery Clinics of North America is covered in *MEDLINE/PubMed* (*Index Medicus*).

Printed and bound by CPI Group (UK) Ltd, Croydon, CR0 4YY

Transferred to digital print 2012

Contributors

CONSULTING EDITOR

J. REGAN THOMAS, MD, FACS
Professor and Chairman, Department of
Otolaryngology, University of Illinois at
Chicago, Chicago, Illinois

EDITORS

RICHARD L. GOODE, MD
Professor Emeritus, Department of
Otolaryngology-Head and Neck Surgery,
Stanford Medical Center, Stanford, California

SAM P. MOST, MD
Professor and Chief, Division of Facial
Plastic and Reconstructive Surgery, Stanford
University School of Medicine, Stanford,
California

AUTHORS

RICHARD A.K. CHAFFOO, MD, FICS, FACS
Associate Clinical Professor, Division of Plastic
Surgery, Department of Surgery, UCSD School
of Medicine, La Jolla; Chief, Division of Plastic
Surgery, Scripps Memorial Hospital, Encinitas,
California

STEVEN H. DAYAN, MD, FACS
Chicago Center for Facial Plastic Surgery;
DeNova Research; Department of
Otolaryngology, University of Illinois at
Chicago, Chicago, Illinois

RICHARD L. GOODE, MD
Professor Emeritus, Department of
Otolaryngology-Head and Neck Surgery,
Stanford Medical Center, Stanford, California

ETHAN B. HANDLER, MD
Chief Resident Surgeon, Department of Head
and Neck Surgery, Kaiser Permanente Medical
Center, Oakland, California

BASIL HASSOUNEH, MD
Department of Otolaryngology-Head & Neck
Surgery, University of Toronto, Toronto;
Department of Clinical Epidemiology and
Biostatistics, McMaster University, Hamilton,
Ontario, Canada

ROBERT M. KELLMAN, MD, FACS
Professor & Chair, Department of
Otolaryngology & Communication Sciences,
Upstate Medical University, State University
of New York, Syracuse, New York

DON O. KIKKAWA, MD, FACS
Professor and Chief, Division of Oculofacial
Plastic and Reconstructive Surgery,
Department of Ophthalmology, University of
California at San Diego, La Jolla, California

BOBBY S. KORN, MD, PhD, FACS
Associate Professor, Division of Oculofacial
Plastic and Reconstructive Surgery,
Department of Ophthalmology, University of
California at San Diego, La Jolla, California

SAMUEL M. LAM, MD, FACS
Director, Lam Institute for Hair Restoration,
Plano, Texas

JESSYKA G. LIGHTHALL, MD
Department of Otolaryngology/Head and
Neck Surgery, Oregon Health and Science
University, Portland, Oregon

LISA M. MORRIS, MD
Department of Otolaryngology &
Communication Sciences, Upstate Medical
University, State University of New York,
Syracuse, New York

SAM P. MOST, MD
Professor and Chief, Division of Facial
Plastic and Reconstructive Surgery, Stanford
University School of Medicine, Stanford,
California

VLADIMIR NEKHENDZY, MD
Clinical Associate Professor of Anesthesia
and Otolaryngology, Director, Stanford Head
and Neck Anesthesia, Advanced Airway
Management Program, Department of
Anesthesiology, Perioperative and Pain
Medicine, Stanford University School of
Medicine, Stanford, California

JAMES P. NEWMAN, MD
Volunteer Associate Professor, Stanford
University, Palo Alto, California

VIJAY K. RAMAIAH, MD
Clinical Instructor, Department of
Anesthesiology, Perioperative and Pain
Medicine, Stanford University School of
Medicine, Stanford, California

CHARLES SHIH, MD
Chief of Facial Plastic and Reconstructive
Surgery, Department of Head and Neck
Surgery, Kaiser Permanente Medical Center,
Oakland, California

TARA SONG, MD
Resident Surgeon, Department of Head and
Neck Surgery, Kaiser Permanente Medical
Center, Oakland, California

JOSHUA B. SUROWITZ, MD
Division of Facial Plastic and Reconstructive
Surgery, Stanford Department of
Otolaryngology/Head and Neck Surgery,
Stanford, California

TOM D. WANG, MD, FACS
Director Facial Plastic & Reconstructive
Surgery, Department of Otolaryngology/Head
& Neck Surgery, Oregon Health and Science
University, Portland, Oregon

KATHERINE M. WHIPPLE, MD
Clinical Instructor, Division of Oculofacial
Plastic and Reconstructive Surgery,
Department of Ophthalmology, University
of California at San Diego, La Jolla, California

CHARLES R. WOODARD, MD
Assistant Professor, Division of
Otolaryngology-Head & Neck Surgery,
Facial Plastic and Reconstructive Surgery,
Duke University Medical Center, Durham,
North Carolina

Contents

Rhytidectomy remains a challenging surgical procedure for even the most experienced aesthetic plastic surgeons. The challenges are compounded by complications that are inherent to this procedure and place added pressure on the doctor-patient relationship. Expectations for both parties are high and the margin for error nil. This article presents a personal approach to the avoidance and management of complications associated with facelift surgery. It presents the author's personal approach as a plastic surgeon in the practice of aesthetic plastic surgery over the past 25 years. Clinical pearls are provided to obtain optimum results in rhytidectomy and limit associated sequelae.

Although office-based anesthesia for facial cosmetic surgery remains remarkably safe, no anesthesia or sedation performed outside the operating room should be considered minor. Proper organization, preparation, and patient selection, close collaboration with the surgeon, and expert and effective anesthesia care will increase patient safety and improve perioperative outcomes and patient satisfaction. This article presents a comprehensive overview of anesthesia in terms of facial plastic surgery procedures, beginning with a broad review of essentials and pitfalls of anesthesia, followed by details of specific anesthetic agents, their administration, mechanism of action, and complications.

This article reviews some basic principles of patient selection for facial plastic surgery. There are patients who are not good candidates, independent of the deformity and the ability of the surgeon. Reasons include subtle and not so subtle psychiatric disorders, unrealistic expectations, lack of communication despite multiple visits, and litigious patients. Complications or suboptimal results are not well handled in these patients and often produce an uncomfortable experience for the surgeon and staff in the postoperative period. These patients are best avoided or should be provided a much longer evaluation period prior to any surgery.

Lasers, injectable fillers, and neurotoxins are widely used in facial restoration and rejuvenation by a variety of practitioners. Although they are less invasive than traditional surgical modalities, they still carry risks for both transient as well as permanent complications. It is paramount for the practitioner to understand these complications, optimize their prevention, and initiate appropriate treatment when they are encountered. This article reviews early, often transient, complications as well as delayed, often prolonged or permanent, complications, with particular focus on prevention and management.

Local flaps are a common reconstructive technique of the head and neck. Consequently, knowledge of fundamental concepts and pitfalls to avoid will reduce surgical complications. These complications result from tension-related, ischemic, hematologic, and infectious causes. This paper seeks to address each of these causes with pearls to accomplish a successful outcome.

This article reviews common complications encountered in the setting of facial trauma. Many complications are the result of the primary injury, and a facial plastic surgeon should be able to quickly identify these to prevent further morbidity. Common pitfalls and controversial topics are presented, as well as an overview of treatment for many complications.

Complications and prevention of complications in brow lift are presented. A discussion of anatomic features of the brow introduces the article in keeping with the focus that a thorough understanding of the anatomy, patient variations, and potential complications is requisite for surgeons performing forehead rejuvenation. The varying approaches to brow lift are discussed. Complications reviewed are bleeding, nerve injury, scarring, alopecia, brow asymmetry, and brow elevation overcorrection or undercorrection.

The goal of this article is to enhance the surgical precision and accuracy of surgeons performing upper and lower eyelid blepharoplasty. The most common blepharoplasty complications are described and how to avoid them is discussed in detail. Complications range from mild to severe and for each, preoperative measures to prevent, perioperative measures to avoid, and postoperative measures to minimize complications are detailed. After reading this article the surgeon should have a greater understanding of blepharoplasty complications and how to best manage and avoid them.

This article provides a concise description of common complications of rhinoplasty, recommendations for avoidance, and corrective techniques. The surgeon must have a comprehensive understanding of nasal anatomy and effects of surgical maneuvers to help avoid complications. Meticulous history, physical examination, and standardized photographic documentation are central to preoperative evaluation and surgical planning for rhinoplasty. Photographic documentation is useful to illustrate preexisting preoperative asymmetries. Appropriate preoperative counseling regarding appropriate postoperative expectations as well as all risks, benefits, and alternatives is critical. Any complications should be openly discussed with the patient.

Prominent ears are a fairly common and emotionally charged facial variation. Both children and adults may suffer a damaged psyche secondary to outside ridicule and self-criticism from ears that "stick out." The external ear anatomy is intricate, with thin skin and resilient cartilage. These underlying characteristics make the ears prone to the overt display of surgical correction. This article details the various acute and chronic complications of otoplasty and includes tips and pearls to help prevent and treat these occurrences.

Adverse reactions and unintended effects can occasionally occur with toxins for cosmetic use, even although they generally have an outstanding safety profile. As the use of fillers becomes increasingly more common, adverse events can be expected to increase as well. This article discusses complication avoidance, addressing appropriate training and proper injection techniques, along with patient selection and patient considerations. In addition to complications, avoidance or amelioration of common adverse events is discussed.

Hair restoration requires a high level of specialized skill on the part of both the surgeon and the assistant team. Recipient-site problems can manifest from either surgeon or assistant error. The surgeon can create an unnatural hairline due to lack of knowledge of natural hair-loss patterns or badly executed recipient sites. He must also be cognizant of how hairs naturally are angled on the scalp to re-create a pattern that appears natural when making recipient sites. Assistants can also greatly contribute to the success or failure of surgery in their task of graft dissection and graft placement.

FACIAL PLASTIC SURGERY CLINICS OF NORTH AMERICA

RELATED INTEREST

Surgery (Oxford), Volume 29, Issue 2, February 2011, Pages 67–9
Management Principles of Common Surgical Complications - *Review Article*
Robin Bhatia

NOW AVAILABLE FOR YOUR iPhone and iPad

Advisory Board to Facial Plastic Surgery Clinics 2013

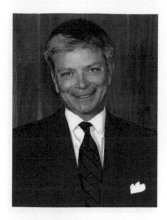
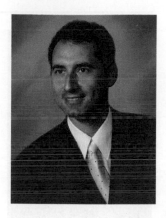
Facial Plastic Surgery Clinics is pleased to introduce the 2012-2013 **Advisory Board**.

Facial Plastic Surgery Clinics is widely available through the media of print, digital e-Reader, online via the Internet, and on iPad and smart phones.

Facial Plastic Surgery Clinics provides professionals access to pertinent point-of-care answers and current clinical information, along with comprehensive background information for deeper understanding.

Readers are welcome to contact the Clinics Editor or Board with comments.

BOARD MEMBERS 2013

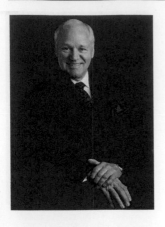

PETER A. ADAMSON, MD

Professor and Head
Division of Facial Plastic and Reconstructive Surgery
Department of Otolaryngology–Head and Neck Surgery
University of Toronto
Toronto, Ontario, Canada

Adamson Cosmetic Facial Surgery
Renaissance Plaza; 150 Bloor Street West; Suite M110
Toronto, Ontario M5S 2X9

416.323.3900
paa@dradamson.com
www.dradamson.com

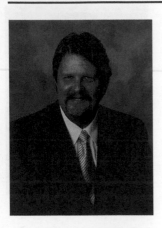

RICK DAVIS, MD

Voluntary Professor
The University of Miami Miller School of Medicine
Miami, Florida

The Center for Facial Restoration
1951 S.W. 172nd Ave; Suite 205
Miramar, Florida 33029

954.442.5191
drd@davisrhinoplasty.com
www.DavisRhinoplasty.com

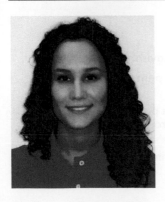

TATIANA DIXON, MD

University of Illinois at Chicago
Resident,
Department of Otolaryngology–Head and Neck Surgery

1855 W. Taylor
Chicago, IL 60612

312.996.6555
TFeuer1@UIC.EDU

STEVEN FAGIEN, MD, FACS

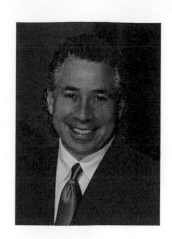

Aesthetic Eyelid Plastic Surgery
660 Glades Road; Suite 210
Boca Raton, Florida 33431

561.393.9898
sfagien@aol.com

GREG KELLER, MD

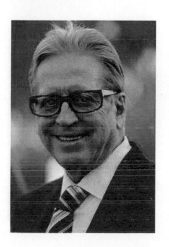

Clinical Professor of Surgery, Head and Neck,
David Geffen School of Medicine,
University of California, Los Angeles;

Keller Facial Plastic Surgery
221 W. Pueblo St. Ste A
Santa Barbara, CA 93105

805.687.6408
faclft@aol.com
www.gregorykeller.com

THEDA C. KONTIS, MD

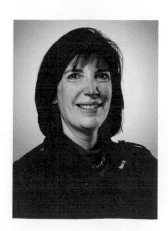

Assistant Professor, Johns Hopkins Hospital
Facial Plastic Surgicenter, Ltd.
1838 Greene Tree Road, Suite 370
Baltimore, MD 21208

410.486.3400
tckontis@aol.com
www.facialplasticsurgerymd.com
www.facial-plasticsurgery.com

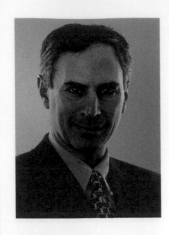

IRA D. PAPEL, MD

Facial Plastic Surgicenter
Associate Professor
The Johns Hopkins University
1838 Greene Tree Road, Suite 370
Baltimore, MD 21208

410.486.3400
idpmd@aol.com
www.facial-plasticsurgery.com

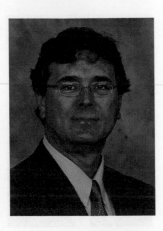

SHERARD A. TATUM, MD

Professor of Otolaryngology and
Pediatrics Cleft and Craniofacial Center
Division of Facial Plastic Surgery
Upstate Medical University
750 E. Adams St.
Syracuse, NY 13210

315.464.4636
TatumS@upstate.edu
www.upstate.edu

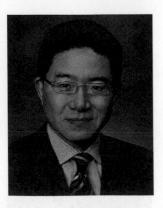

TOM D. WANG, MD

Professor
Facial Plastic and Reconstructive Surgery
Oregon Health & Science University
3181 Southwest Sam Jackson Park Road
Portland, OR 97239

503.494.5678
wangt@ohsu.edu
www.ohsu.edu/drtomwang

Preface
Complications in Facial Plastic Surgery

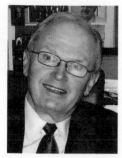 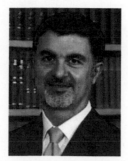

Richard L. Goode, MD   Sam P. Most, MD
Editors

Writing about complications in facial plastic surgery is not what most surgeons want to do. We would rather write about how we perform our surgical procedures or how we solve certain surgical challenges with innovative approaches resulting in good outcomes.

To be comfortable in writing about complications, how to avoid them, and how to treat them—the topics addressed in this issue of the *Facial Plastic Surgery Clinics of North America*—requires experience and confidence. We feel we have assembled an outstanding group to address this important subject and thank them for their contributions.

Richard L. Goode, MD
Department of Otolaryngology–Head and
Neck Surgery
Stanford Medical Center
801 Welch Road
Stanford, CA 94305, USA

Sam P. Most, MD
Division of Facial Plastic and
Reconstructive Surgery
Stanford University School of Medicine
801 Welch Road
Stanford, CA 94305, USA

E-mail addresses:
rgoode@ohns.stanford.edu (R.L. Goode)
smost@ohns.stanford.edu (S.P. Most)

Facial Plast Surg Clin N Am 21 (2013) xiii
http://dx.doi.org/10.1016/j.fsc.2013.07.004
1064-7406/13/$ – see front matter © 2013 Published by Elsevier Inc.

facialplastic.theclinics.com

Complications in Facelift Surgery: Avoidance and Management

Richard A.K. Chaffoo, MD, FACS, FICS[a,b,*]

KEYWORDS

• Facelift • Rhytidectomy • Facelift complications • Cosmetic surgery • Facial rejuvenation

KEY POINTS

- Facelift surgery yields high satisfaction for most patients who have aesthetic surgery and most women and men who seek facial rejuvenation surgery are generally well adjusted psychologically and have realistic expectations.
- Complications related to facelift surgery can be divided into 3 main areas: preoperative assessment and surgical planning, intraoperative surgical maneuvers, and postoperative care.
- A methodical operative plan based on the patient's aesthetic deformities executed in a meticulous manner helps to limit intraoperative complications.
- Of all complications related to rhytidectomy, the so-called "done look" is perhaps the most common and most difficult (or impossible) to correct.
- A thorough history and physical elicit evidence of prior complications associated with anesthesia and surgery.
- Hematoma formation typically occurs within the first 24 hours following surgery, and is the most common postoperative complication.

INTRODUCTION

Rhytidectomy continues to be one of the most common aesthetic procedures performed by plastic surgeons, as reported in the annual statistics by the American Society for Aesthetic Plastic Surgery. It consistently ranks within the top 10 aesthetic surgical procedures performed in the United States each year, with more than 100,000 performed in 2010, an increase of 28.5% since 1997.[1] Despite widespread public acceptance of aesthetic surgery, complications related to facelift surgery persist. This article reviews the common complications and proposes strategies to reduce or eliminate them wherever possible.

Complications related to facelift surgery can be divided into 3 main areas: preoperative assessment and surgical planning, intraoperative surgical maneuvers, and postoperative care. Although some complications are unavoidable and unforeseen with any surgical procedure, patients are less forgiving and tolerant of those associated with an aesthetic surgical procedure.

Some complications can be avoided during the preoperative evaluation. A thorough history and physical elicit evidence of prior complications associated with anesthesia and surgery. Easy bruising or postoperative bleeding should alert the surgeon that a coagulation work-up may be indicated. Patients are instructed to avoid the use of aspirin and nonsteroidal antiinflammatory drugs for at least 2 weeks before surgery. Smoking must be discontinued for at least 4 weeks before surgery. All herbal preparations, vitamins, and homeopathic treatments should also be avoided for 2 weeks before surgery because of the risk of postoperative bleeding and intraoperative anesthetic complications, including arrhythmias (**Box 1**).

Disclosures: None.
a Division of Plastic Surgery, Department of Surgery, UCSD School of Medicine, La Jolla, CA, USA; b Division of Plastic Surgery, Scripps Memorial Hospital, Encinitas, CA, USA
* Suite 480, Scripps Ximed Medical Building, 9850 Genesee Avenue, La Jolla, CA 92037.
E-mail address: drc@drchaffoo.com

Facial Plast Surg Clin N Am 21 (2013) 551–558
http://dx.doi.org/10.1016/j.fsc.2013.07.007
1064-7406/13/$ – see front matter © 2013 Elsevier Inc. All rights reserved.

Box 1
Herbal supplements to avoid before surgery

Dong quai, *Ginkgo biloba*, St. John's wort (all types)

Echinacea, ginseng, valerian

Ephedra, glucosamine, vitamin C (>2000 mg daily)

Feverfew, goldenseal, vitamin E (>400 mg daily)

Fish oils (omega-3 fatty acids)

Garlic, licorice

Kava

Licorice

Chemotherapeutic agents and oral steroid usage can alter wound healing and must be discontinued several weeks before elective surgery. In addition, close communication and clearance with the patient's primary care physician and specialist is needed to determine suitability for elective aesthetic surgery.

The initial consultation must include a thorough assessment of the patient's signs of facial aging. This assessment includes an evaluation of skin tone and laxity, facial rhytids, dyschromia, previous facial scars, skin atrophy, telangiectasia (worsened with facial surgery), and presence or absence of facial fat. Facial fat is important in that care must be taken during flap elevation to avoid perforation of the superficial muscular aponeurotic system (SMAS) and facial nerve injury. Furthermore, aggressive liposuction in such patients may result in visible and/or palpable contour irregularities of the face and neck.

Facial nerve paresis or paralysis must be documented and demonstrated to the patient. Submalar hollowing, microgenia, and facial asymmetry need to be recognized and discussed with the patient. Submandibular gland ptosis, low-riding hyoid, and platysmal bands are also documented. Deep neck rhytids, perioral rhytids, and nasolabial folds are unaffected by rhytidectomy so alternative treatment plans can be discussed at the initial consultation. The hairline needs to be inspected carefully. The position of the frontal and temporal hairlines should be noted along with any alopecia.

Patient expectations and goals should be discussed. It may be possible to identify a particularly difficult or manipulative patient before the consultation based on the patient's interactions with the office staff. The aesthetic deformities must be correctly identified during this consultation, and the surgeon needs to develop an appropriate surgical plan to manage each deformity. It is paramount that an open and honest dialogue occurs between surgeon and patient as to the deformities that will be improved at the time of rhytidectomy. Realistic goals need to be agreed on with the patient in advance because a thorough preoperative discussion and explanation of the limitations of rhytidectomy are interpreted by the patient as a sign of a meticulous and ethical plastic surgeon. If this discussion occurs only after surgery, it is viewed with suspicion by the patient and interpreted as making excuses for an outcome that the patient perceives as suboptimal.

An evaluation of the skin is critical in the aesthetic analysis of every patient. Extensive skin laxity may alert the surgeon that a minor touch-up or further skin excision may be needed several months after the initial rhytidectomy, especially in elderly patients and those with prior extensive sun exposure or steroid use. Facial dyschromia and telangiectasia can be exacerbated by rhytidectomy.

Facial asymmetry is common in patients who present for aesthetic surgery. This asymmetry may be the result of, among other things, prior facial surgery, trauma, facial nerve injury, soft tissue atrophy, skeletal abnormalities, brow ptosis, or alopecia. It is necessary to point out this asymmetry to the patient in a mirror and explain that it may persist after rhytidectomy. Submalar atrophy may respond to soft tissue augmentation performed at the same time as the rhytidectomy, especially in the case of fat transfer. Microgenia can be corrected concurrently and creates a more youthful jaw and neck contour.

Submandibular gland ptosis is not improved by most rhytidectomy techniques and may even be accentuated with aggressive liposuction in the submandibular area. This limitation needs to be discussed with the patient at the initial consultation. Techniques are available to remove the submandibular glands causing this ptosis but the author (an otolaryngologist and plastic surgeon) does not advocate such an approach. Such surgery can result in significant morbidity, including facial nerve, lingual nerve, and hypoglossal nerve injury and hemorrhage from the facial and lingual arteries, which might compromise the patient's airway.

Platysmal laxity should be noted at the consultation and a surgical plan formulated to improve this deformity. In general, platysmal laxity can be improved with plication. However, overly aggressive surgery, including extensive subplatysmal lipectomy and digastric muscle resection, can produce an unnatural and overly operated-on appearance to the neck, including witch's chin, cobra deformity, and a skeletonized and cadaveric neck, which does not look rejuvenated.

It is important to evaluate the patient's hairline and look for evidence of alopecia. The present position of the temporal and mastoid hairlines needs to be respected in the design of any rhytidectomy incisions. The temporal hairline must not be elevated or narrowed as the result of a poorly designed incision. The upper end of the rhytidectomy incision should be placed along and parallel to the lower end of the temporal hairline and should not extend above the upper edge of the pinna. If it does, the temporal hairline is raised and narrowed, compromising the final aesthetic result and making reconstruction of this valuable landmark difficult. Hairline incisions in the mastoid and post auricular area should be avoided because they often result in hypopigmented and quite obvious scars that prevent the patient from wearing her hair up, which might expose them. If it is necessary to extend the incision behind the ear, then it is prudent to continue it into the hair-bearing scalp.

INTRAOPERATIVE COMPLICATIONS
Positioning and Preparation

Careful patient positioning following anesthesia and before surgery improves patient visibility and outcome and reduces complications. Suturing the endotracheal tube to the lower central incisors stabilizes the airway and avoids the use of tape on the face, with its subsequent distortion of surrounding structures. The head is positioned in a small donut for occipital support and the arms tucked at the patient's sides. It is sometimes helpful to place a small roll between the shoulder blades to extend the neck adequately. The eyes are lubricated, taped, and checked frequently throughout the procedure to prevent corneal drying. Local anesthesia is infiltrated before the surgical prep to allow the epinephrine effect to occur by the time of the surgical incision. The hair is prepped in the surgical field because it is an important aesthetic landmark but may require rubber bands to keep it off the field. Cotton balls are placed in the ear canals to reduce blood pooling here.

Incision and Flap Dissection

The skin incision is created with a #15 blade and the skin flaps elevated a short distance with the knife and single-toothed Addison forceps. Next, the flaps are first elevated using double skin hooks and then Deaver retractors to avoid trauma to them. The flaps are then elevated with tenotomy scissors for about 2–3 cm while the assistant retracts the skin medially. The overhead surgical lights are shone on the outer surface of the skin flaps and not directly into the surgical field for transillumination. This method allows the surgeon to ensure the proper plane of dissection of the skin flaps. The light should shine through the flaps, indicating that a small amount of fat is on the undersurface of the flaps, the so-called peau d'orange effect. If the light becomes dim or absent, it indicates that the surgeon is in too deep a surgical plane and adjustment needs to be done to avoid perforation of the SMAS. Deeper dissection may result in inadvertent injury to the parotid fascia and underlying gland, increasing the possibility of parotid fistula.

After the initial 2–3 cm of dissection with tenotomy scissors, the flap dissection continues with flat, long-bladed facelift scissors by bluntly raising 2 tunnels and connecting them under direct vision. The dissection of the flap continues along the mandible to release both the masseteric cutaneous and mandibular cutaneous ligaments (**Figs. 1** and **2**).

Parotid duct injury

Injury to the parotid duct may occur along the anterior border of the masseter on a line from the external auditory canal to the upper lip. If it is injured, the distal end of the duct is cannulated with a small catheter and passed retrograde into the field and then passed into the proximal severed end. The duct can be sutured with 6-0 nylon sutures and the catheter left in place for about 2 weeks.

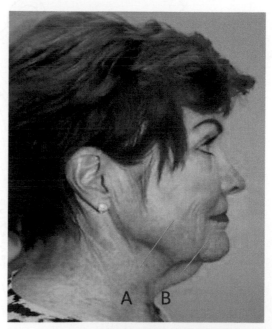

Fig. 1. Preoperative rhytidectomy. (A) Masseteric cutaneous ligament. (B) Mandibular cutaneous ligament.

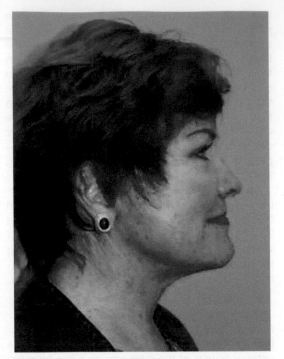

Fig. 2. Postoperative rhytidectomy.

Facial nerve branch injury

Injury of branches of the facial nerve can occur during flap dissection if the dissection is too deep. If recognized during the surgery, the nerve can be repaired with 6-0 nylon sutures after identification of the distal severed branch by nerve stimulation and a lack of paralytic anesthetic agents. The temporal branch is most vulnerable anterior to the temporal hairline so dissection here must be superficial with observation of the overlying hair follicles in the skin flap to ensure proper plane position. Marginal mandibular and cervical branch injuries are possible if the dissection below the mandibular border extends beneath the platysma. Bipolar cautery is helpful in areas where the facial nerve branches are superficial, such as the temporal and cheek regions.

Auricular nerve and jugular vein injury

The posterior neck flap dissection must be done superficially but without buttonholing the skin flap. Care is taken to avoid exposing the fascia overlying the sternocleidomastoid muscle and risking injury to the great auricular nerve and accompanying external jugular vein. If injured, direct repair of nerve and suture ligature of vein should be undertaken.

Spinal accessory nerve injury

More posteriorly, injury to the spinal accessory nerve can occur if the dissection becomes too deep. A good superficial landmark to keep in mind is Erb's point (**Fig. 3**), which is a point along the posterior border of the sternocleidomastoid

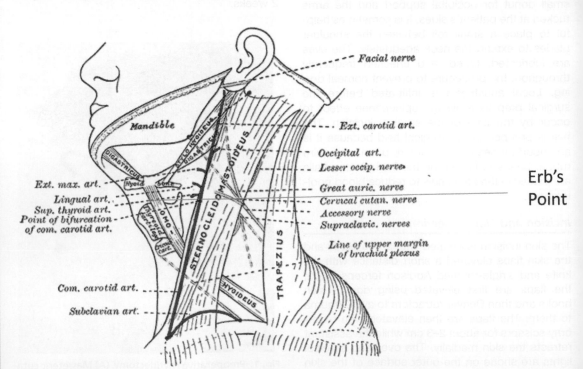

Fig. 3. Erb point.

muscle midway between the mastoid and clavicle. It can be estimated by drawing a horizontal line from the thyroid notch to the posterior border of the sternocleidomastoid muscle. It is the point from which the nerve roots of C5 and C6 converge. It is also the location of the greater auricular nerve. Most importantly, the spinal accessory nerve exits from the posterior border of the muscle within 2 cm superior or inferior to the Erb's point.

Jowl Liposuction

Once flap elevation is completed, direct liposuction of the jowls can be performed gently with a 1-mm or 2-mm liposuction cannula keeping the open end of the cannula down away from the undersurface of the flap to avoid contour deformities. Liposuction must be done gently to avoid paresis of the marginal mandibular nerve. Liposuction posterior to the mandibular angle helps define this area and create a more youthful jawline.

SMAS Plication

Plication of the SMAS is done using 4-0 Mersilene sutures, with care taken to avoid penetration of the parotid fascia and parotid gland. The plication should include just the SMAS or a parotid fistula may occur, resulting in postoperative gustatory swelling and erythema, which may necessitate wound exploration and suture removal. If the plication results in tissue elevation, these irregularities should be carefully trimmed flush with the surrounding tissue to avoid noticeable contour deformities after surgery. The decision to use a drain is made now based on the appearance of the operative field. If the field appears wet, small round drains are placed through a small stab incision in the postauricular sulcus and typically removed the following day. The drains are useful to reduce postoperative edema and ecchymosis in such situations but not to reduce hematoma formation.

Skin Excision and Wound Closure

Meticulous hemostasis is paramount at this point before skin removal and wound closure. Pinpoint bipolar cautery is useful and reduces trauma to the underlying facial nerve branches, thereby limiting postoperative facial nerve neurapraxia. Skin flaps are redraped and checked for signs of vascular compromise. Excess skin is removed and closure performed first at the temporal hairline. Most tension on the flaps occurs here because of the lifting nature of the flap redraping versus posterior pulling with its subsequent windswept look. Several 4-0 monocryl sutures are placed in the subcutaneous/deep dermal position.

Further skin excision is done down to just above the tragus with no tension to avoid distortion of the auricle. All further skin excision must be conservative. The tragal flaps are conservatively defatted and conservatively trimmed to eliminate any widening of the ear canal. The skin around the ear lobes is carefully removed so that the ear lobes are free with no tension. The same conservative approach is used in the postauricular sulcus. Skin closure is with interrupted 5-0 monocryl dermal sutures and 5-0 nylon skin sutures, except 5-0 fast-absorbing gut for the tragal closure. The submental incision is closed last, with final inspection of the submental area for hemostasis.

Immediate Postoperative Procedures

Placement of a compressive dressing for the first 24 hours after surgery may reduce the extent of edema and ecchymosis. Fluffs are placed around each ear for padding and to prevent inadvertent folding over of the external ears. Kerlix and bias are wrapped around the face and neck as a figure-of-eight dressing. Communication is important between the surgeon and anesthesiologist to avoid excess coughing and straining during extubation, which could cause hematoma formation. The head of the bed is elevated with the knees flexed and ice applied to the central face in the recovery room. Postoperative nausea is monitored and treated promptly in the recovery room and during the first several days after surgery with antiemetic agents to reduce ecchymosis.

POSTOPERATIVE COMPLICATIONS
Hematoma

Hematoma formation typically occurs within the first 24 hours following surgery, and is the most common postoperative complication, occurring in 3% to 8% of cases according to multiple studies.[2–6]

Before discharge, the dressings are inspected and flaps viewed with a flashlight while lifting up the Kerlix wrap from each cheek. If there is significant pain or asymmetric swelling, the dressings are immediately removed and the flaps inspected. The patient is returned to the operating room if a hematoma is discovered because further delay places the flaps at risk, and an expanding hematoma can compromise the patient's airway if not managed immediately. The incision is opened, clots evacuated, bleeding controlled, and the incisions closed over an active drain. Early and prompt intervention reduces the risk of further vascular compromise to an already compromised flap.

Infection

Infection is unusual following rhytidectomy but may occur as the result of a stitch abscess or, more rarely, a suture passed through the tragal cartilage. The offending suture(s) should be removed and local wound care with an antimicrobial ointment often clears the problem. Significant erythema and tenderness to the auricular cartilage warrants oral antibiotics to cover *Staphylococcus*, *Streptococcus*, and *Pseudomonas* to prevent permanent cartilage damage.

Nerve Injury

Nerve injury is rare but has been reported at rates from 0.7% to 2.5% in large series.[7] If noted during surgery, primary repair results in the best outcome. Mild facial paresis is usually temporary but may persist for 12 hours after surgery, caused by the prolonged duration of local anesthetic agents or edema of the nerve. Permanent nerve injuries may involve sensory and motor nerves. The great auricular nerve is the most frequently injured sensory nerve and results in numbness. If the nerve is repaired during surgery, return of sensation is common but may be delayed for 12 to 18 months and result in localized areas of persistent anesthesia. The temporal branch is the most frequently injured motor nerve in most series; the delay is usually temporary, reported as 0.8% in a review of more than 12,000 rhytidectomies. Permanent injury was noted in 0.1% of the cases in this large retrospective study. Temporal nerve injury may resolve within 18 to 24 months of onset but the resultant asymmetric brow can be improved with careful use of paralytic agents like Botox or Dysport on the non-paralyzed side. If the forehead paralysis is permanent, treatment is dictated by the extent of the subsequent deformity and disability. Mild asymmetry is best managed by the paralytic agents mentioned earlier, whereas significant brow ptosis may require a brow lift on the affected side.

Other nerve injuries may include marginal mandibular, zygomatic, buccal, or cervical branches of the facial nerve, and permanent damage was less than 1% in a large study.[7] Temporary injury is dictated by paresis versus paralysis and length of time since surgery. Permanent injury is likely if no return of function occurs after 2 years. Long-term management of paralysis depends on the branch injured, subsequent deformity, and functional deficits.

Systemic Complications

Major systemic complications are unusual in patients undergoing facelift surgery, reported as 0.1% in a large facelift survey by the American Society of Plastic Surgeons. Major complications included deep vein thrombosis (DVT), pulmonary embolism, stroke, blood transfusions, major anesthetic complications, and death. A more recent report by the American Society for Aesthetic Plastic Surgery discussed a single center's experience with venous thromboembolism in which 630 patients underwent rhytidectomy and 3 cases of DVT were identified.[8] Risk factors included operative time more than 5 hours and combining rhytidectomy with other procedures. DVT diagnosis was established by ultrasound and confirmed by computed tomography. Patients were admitted and received anticoagulation therapy followed by warfarin for 6 months. All patients recovered with full resolution of their symptoms.

Skin Slough

Skin slough is a rare occurrence following rhytidectomy. The skin flaps are monitored closely during the postoperative course. Vascular compromise is usually noted in the periauricular region and may appear as a distinct area of ecchymosis. Local application of nitropaste or DMSO 2 to 3 times daily may be beneficial to reduce the chance of full-thickness skin loss. More often, there is a superficial epidermolysis that heals uneventfully. Nevertheless, the area of concern is allowed to demarcate fully into an eschar before conservative debridement is done in the office. The debrided area is protected with an antimicrobial ointment until secondary healing has occurred. Excision of scars and closure are delayed until full maturation of the wound and scars has occurred to prevent further compromise of the flaps and ultimate aesthetic result.

Scarring

Noticeable scars are unusual following a well-designed and well-executed facelift. Hypertrophic scars are injected with a dilute concentration of Kenalog 2% to 5% every 6 weeks once noted, along with the use of silicone sheeting or gels. Persistent scars may respond to pulsed dye laser therapy if resistant to the aforementioned measures and usually require multiple treatments. The laser also reduces the telangiectasia that occurs following prolonged steroid injections. Hypopigmented scars are most common along the posterior hairline when incisions have been placed along the hairline instead of behind it. These scars can be reduced by medical tattooing or the insertion of hair grafts into the scar.

Alopecia

Alopecia occurs following damage to the hair follicles from electrocautery, excess traction of tension on the skin flaps, and inadvertent elevation or elimination of the temporal hair tuft and temporal hairline. Temporary loss may be shortened with the use of topical minoxidil. Permanent alopecia requires the insertion of single-hair follicular units into the areas of alopecia or the replacement or lowering of the temporal hairline. Definitive hair replacement surgery should be delayed until it is certain that the loss is permanent, which often requires 12 months to ascertain.

Contour Deformities

Contour deformities are common immediately after rhytidectomy. Most of these are temporary and related to postoperative edema and ecchymosis and occur in the preauricular and submental regions. As the swelling subsides, most of these resolve, and resolution may be hastened with gentle local digital massage. Persistent contour deformities may be seen for several months and require no further treatment. If localized areas of depression persist after 6 to 12 months, they can be improved by injections of dermal fillers or fat.

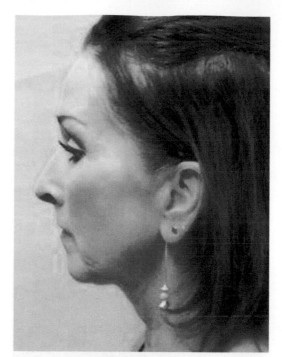

Fig. 4. Preoperative rhytidectomy.

SUMMARY

Despite the complexities and challenges, facelift surgery continues to yield high satisfaction for most patients who have aesthetic surgery. Most women and men who seek facial rejuvenation surgery are generally well adjusted psychologically and have realistic goals and expectations. As an aesthetic plastic surgeon ages and matures, so does his patient base and community reputation. The natural outcome is for surgeons to see more patients for facial rejuvenation when they are seasoned surgeons, which is fortunate for both patient and surgeon.

Complications related to rhytidectomy are an inevitable outcome of a busy aesthetic plastic surgery practice. It is imperative that the surgeon constantly strives to reduce the incidence and severity by a proactive approach. The initial history and physical examination must be overseen by the responsible surgeon to elicit information that might be overlooked by a nurse or other office assistant. The patient's demeanor and interaction with the surgeon may either reinforce that of the office staff or contradict it. When in doubt, it is always prudent to defer surgery and allow the patient to choose another, less fortunate colleague.

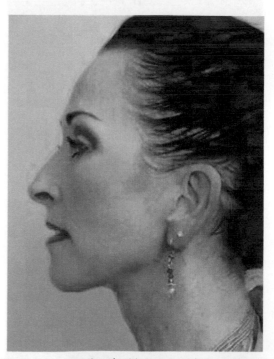

Fig. 5. Postoperative rhytidectomy with normal periauricular architecture and preserved temporal tuft.

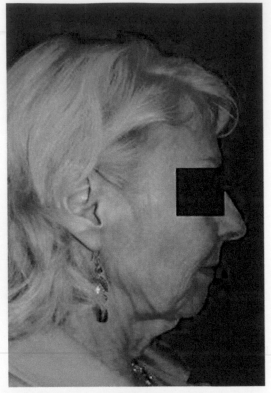

Fig. 6. Preoperative rhytidectomy.

A methodical operative plan based on the patient's aesthetic deformities executed in a meticulous manner helps to limit intraoperative complications. Vigilant postoperative care by the surgeon and trained staff are vital to recognize and treat any postoperative complications. Once a complication is recognized, the surgeon must maintain good communication with the patient along with frequent office visits to manage the subsequent physical and psychological effects.

Overall, what patients fear most is the so-called "done look." Of all the complications related to rhytidectomy, this is perhaps the most common and most difficult (or impossible) to correct. All patients have seen examples of this in their communities, and it is what they most fear. The hallmarks of this include an overly stretched, pulled, or tightened face with distortion of the mouth. The hairline is distorted or raised and scars are evident around the ears and hairline. The results are neither youthful nor aesthetic. In men, the end result is feminization of the face, which might be why men are initially more reluctant than women to consider rhytidectomy. Patients are relieved when assured that great plastic surgery is natural looking and often goes unnoticed by family and friends (**Figs. 4–7**).

REFERENCES

1. Cosmetic Surgery National Data Bank Statistics, 2010. American Society for Aesthetic Plastic Surgery.
2. Leist FD, Masson JK, Erich JB. A review of 324 rhytidectomies, emphasizing complications and patient dissatisfaction. Plast Reconstr Surg 1977;59:525.
3. Conway H. Analysis of 25 consecutive rhytidectomies. N Y State J Med 1967;67:790.
4. McDowell A. Effective practical steps to avoid complications in facelifting. Plast Reconstr Surg 1972;50:563.
5. McGregor M, et al. Complications of facelifting. In: Symposium of aesthetic surgery of the face, eyelid, and breast, vol. 4. St Louis (MO): Mosby; 1972. p. 58–64.
6. Baker TJ, Gordon HL. Complications of rhytidectomy. Plast Reconstr Surg 1967;40:31.
7. Matarasso A. National plastic surgery survey: face lift techniques and complications. Plast Reconstr Surg 2000;106:1185–95.
8. Abboushi N, Yezhelyev M, Symbas J, et al. Facelift complications and the risk of venous thromboembolism: a single center's experience. Aesthet Surg J 2012;32(4):413–20.

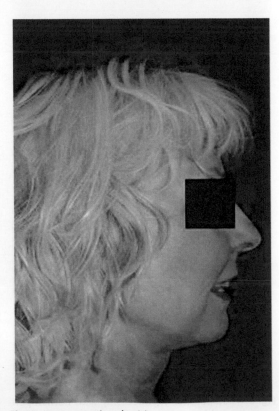

Fig. 7. Postoperative rhytidectomy.

Prevention of Perioperative and Anesthesia-Related Complications in Facial Cosmetic Surgery

Vladimir Nekhendzy, MD[a],*, Vijay K. Ramaiah, MD[b]

KEYWORDS

- Anesthesia complications • Ambulatory surgery • Cosmetic surgery complications

KEY POINTS

- The essential anesthesia requirements for facial cosmetic surgery include a quiet, clear surgical field, absence of patient movement, nonstimulating emergence from anesthesia, a rapid return of consciousness and protective airway reflexes, prevention of postoperative nausea and vomiting, and fast-tracking patients for discharge.
- Facial cosmetic surgical procedures performed under sedation (monitored anesthesia care [MAC]) require extra vigilance and close cooperation between the surgeon and the anesthesiologist. Respiratory depression and rapidly ensuing upper airway obstruction caused by either absolute or relative overdose of sedative or opioid drugs can occur at any time, and may be missed if monitoring is inadequate. Patients with obstructive sleep apnea (OSA) are particularly prone to these life-threatening upper airway-related complications.
- Outpatient anesthesia practice is typically repetitive and predictable, and is therefore uniquely suited to protocol-driven practice improvement.
- Comprehensive surgical safety checklists constitute an essential safeguard, drastically decreasing the number of perioperative complications, reducing health care costs, and improving overall quality of patient care, even when the baseline standard of care is high.

GENERAL CONSIDERATIONS

The volume of cosmetic surgery in the United States continues to grow rapidly: more than 1.6 million surgeries were performed in 2011 alone, an increase of almost 75% since 1997.[1] More than 80% of cosmetic surgeries are performed on the outpatient basis, and 60% in office facilities,[1] typically demonstrating very low rates of perioperative mortality and complications, not exceeding 0.002% and 0.7%, respectively.[2–7] Despite such an excellent safety profile, data from Coldiron and colleagues'[8] 3-year prospective audit of office-based surgical incidents in Florida suggest that facial cosmetic surgery patients may be at a higher anesthetic risk: all (albeit rare) deaths in these patients were anesthesia related, and as much as half of all major anesthetic complications (cardiovascular instability, hypoxia, respiratory failure, and so forth) were observed in this patient category.[8] Analysis of the 2011 American Society for Aesthetic Plastic Surgery National Data Bank

[a] Stanford Head and Neck Anesthesia, Advanced Airway Management Program, Department of Anesthesiology, Perioperative and Pain Medicine, Stanford University School of Medicine, 300 Pasteur Drive, Stanford, CA 94305, USA; [b] Department of Anesthesiology, Perioperative and Pain Medicine, Stanford University School of Medicine, 300 Pasteur Drive, Stanford, CA 94305, USA
* Corresponding author. Department of Anesthesiology, Perioperative and Pain Medicine, Stanford University Medical Center, Room H3580, 300 Pasteur Drive, Stanford, CA 94305-5640.
E-mail address: nek@stanford.edu

Facial Plast Surg Clin N Am 21 (2013) 559–577
http://dx.doi.org/10.1016/j.fsc.2013.07.011
1064-7406/13/$ – see front matter © 2013 Elsevier Inc. All rights reserved.

Statistics[1] conservatively places the number of facial cosmetic surgical and nonsurgical procedures (eg, face lift, rhinoplasty, blepharoplasty, skin resurfacing and rejuvenation) that would require general anesthesia or various degrees of intraoperative sedation at more than 600,000 annually, thus defining the population at risk.

Structural Recommendations and Guidelines

Reducing perioperative risk and the incidence of complications in office-based cosmetic surgery is a multifaceted task (**Box 1**), and starts with the top-down approach that introduces certain structural recommendations and guidelines. The anesthesiologist (and the surgeon) should follow the provisions of the American Society of Anesthesiologists (ASA) Guidelines for Ambulatory Anesthesia and Surgery, the ASA Guidelines for Office-Based Surgery, the ASA Standards for Basic Anesthetic Monitoring, and the ASA Standards for Postanesthesia Care,[9] to ensure that the quality of patient care will meet hospital-based standards.

Some of the essential requirements for patient safety in the office-based surgical setting are[10–15]:

- Accreditation of the facility by either the American Association for Accreditation of Ambulatory Surgical Facilities, the Accreditation Association for Ambulatory Health Care, or the Joint Commission
- Proper patient and procedure selection
- Availability of essential anesthesia and resuscitative equipment, including malignant hyperthermia cart and difficult airway equipment
- Existence of emergency protocols and patient transfer agreements
- Education and training of office personnel

Box 1
Perioperative risk reduction: general considerations

- Accredited surgical facility
- Top-down approach to assure compliance with American Society of Anesthesiologists guidelines and presence of established policies and procedures
- Bottom-up approach with quality improvement and personnel training
- Presence of expert anesthesiologist and surgeon with appropriate knowledge and experience in office-based surgery
- A team approach to patient care
- Safety checklists

Solutions to Identified Problems

It is equally important for the surgeon and anesthesiologist to have an effective bottom-up approach to office-based patient care, ensuring proper documentation and analysis of complications and adverse events, and the development of solutions to the identified problems.[7] Outpatient anesthesia practice is typically repetitive and predictable, and is therefore uniquely suited to protocol-driven practice improvement.[15]

Surgical Safety Checklists

Comprehensive surgical safety checklists constitute another safeguard, drastically decreasing the number of perioperative complications, reducing health care costs, and improving overall quality of patient care, even when the baseline standard of care is high.[13,16,17] For office-based surgery, implementation of a checklist developed by the Institute for Safety in Office-Based Surgery (**Fig. 1**)[18] has resulted in a 6-fold decrease in the incidence of perioperative complications.[19]

PERIOPERATIVE AND ANESTHETIC MANAGEMENT

Anesthetic management of patients undergoing facial cosmetic surgery presents unique challenges to the anesthesiologist. The absent or limited anesthesia backup, inadequate ancillary support, lack of anesthesia equipment, variability of monitoring modalities, and cramped and unfamiliar environment may all make the delivery of anesthesia care in the office-based setting difficult.[14,20]

To provide safe and effective anesthesia care, the anesthesiologist should be experienced with the office-based surgery, serve as a competent consultant for proper patient selection and preparation, understand anesthesia objectives for facial cosmetic surgical procedures, be well versed with total intravenous anesthesia (TIVA) and administering effective sedation without immediate access to the patient's airway, and possess some of the unique techniques of advanced airway management.

Anesthesia Objectives

The essential anesthesia requirements for facial cosmetic surgery include a quiet, clear surgical field, absence of patient movement, nonstimulating emergence from anesthesia, a rapid return of consciousness and protective airway reflexes, prevention of postoperative nausea and vomiting (PONV), and fast-tracking patients for discharge.

Maintenance of a clear surgical field is extremely important owing to the high vascularity of the

Introduction	Setting	Operation	Before discharge	Satisfaction
Preoperative encounter; with practitioner and patient	Before patient in procedure room; with practitioner and personnel	Before sedation/analgesia; with practitioner and personnel*	On arrival to recovery area; with practitioner and personnel	Completed post-procedure; with practitioner and patient
Patient Patient medically optimized for the procedure? ☐ Yes ☐ No, and plan for optimization made	Emergency equipment check complete (e.g. airway, AED, code cart, MH kit)? ☐ Yes	Patient identity, procedure, and consent confirmed? ☐ Yes	Assessment for pain? ☐ Yes	Unanticipated events documented? ☐ Yes
Does patient have DVT risk factors? ☐ Yes, and prophylaxis plans arranged ☐ No	EMS availability confirmed? ☐ Yes	Is the site marked and side identified? ☐ Yes ☐ N/A	Assessment for nausea/vomiting? ☐ Yes	Patient satisfaction assessed? ☐ Yes
Procedure Procedure complexity and sedation/analgesia reviewed? ☐ Yes	Oxygen source and suction checked? ☐ Yes	DVT prophylaxis provided? ☐ Yes ☐ N/A Antibiotic prophylaxis administered within 60 minutes prior to procedure? ☐ Yes ☐ N/A	Recovery personnel available? ☐ Yes *Prior to discharge:* *(with personnel and patient)*	Provider satisfaction assessed? ☐ Yes
NPO instructions given? ☐ Yes	Anticipated duration ≤ 6 hours? ☐ Yes ☐ No, but personnel, monitoring, and equipment available	Essential imaging displayed? ☐ Yes ☐ N/A *Practitioner confirms verbally:* ☐ Local anesthetic toxicity precautions	Discharge criteria achieved? ☐ Yes Patient education and instructions provided? ☐ Yes	
Escort and post-procedure plans reviewed? ☐ Yes		☐ Patient monitoring (per institutional protocol) ☐ Anticipated critical events addressed with team ☐ Each member of the team has been addressed by name and is ready to proceed	Plan for post-discharge follow-up? ☐ Yes Escort confirmed? ☐ Yes	

Fig. 1. Safety checklist for office-based surgery. (*From* The Institute for Safety in Office-Based Surgery (ISOBS). Safety checklist for office-based surgery. Available at: http://isobsurgery.org/wp-content/uploads/2012/03/safety-checklist.jpg. Accessed August 26, 2013; with permission.)

operated areas, where even a small amount of bleeding can have a significant impact on intraoperative exposure. The use of moderate controlled hypotension by the anesthesiologist (see later discussion), and epinephrine-supplemented infiltrative local anesthesia by the surgeon improve both hemostasis and visibility.

Absence of patient movement is required for preventing iatrogenic surgical injury during the delicate parts of the procedure. If general anesthesia is used, deeper anesthetic planes may be necessary to avoid sudden patient motor responses, as intraoperative neuromuscular blockade (NMB) is usually avoided. It is also important for the anesthesiologist to maintain situational awareness in the crowded operating room (OR) environment, to avoid any inadvertent action that may result in accidental movement of the OR table.

Smooth emergence from anesthesia, devoid of patient straining, bucking, and coughing, is essential for avoiding the formation of hematoma, which may require surgical drainage or reexploration, especially after rhytidectomy.[10] Avoidance of PONV is equally important in this regard, and will also reduce the recovery time and the incidence of unanticipated hospital admissions.[10,21]

Assuring a rapid emergence and return of consciousness as well as protective airway reflexes is critical, as supporting the patient's airway with mask ventilation after facial cosmetic surgery will either be difficult (eg, rhytidectomy) or impossible without jeopardizing the cosmetic surgical results (eg, rhinoplasty).

Provision of anesthesia care aimed at fast-tracking patients for discharge is dictated by the overwhelmingly outpatient nature of the facial cosmetic surgical procedures, and by economic considerations of office-based surgery.

A high degree of cooperation with the surgeon is essential to ensure consensus regarding anesthesia objectives, other unique perioperative considerations for a specific procedure, and expectations about patient comfort and satisfaction.[22]

Patient Selection and Preparation

Preoperative risk assessment should take into account the type of facial cosmetic surgery to be performed, and the patient's health status.[22,23] Most patients presenting for facial cosmetic surgery are either completely healthy (ASA physical status I) or have a mild, controlled systemic disease (ASA physical status II). However, a variety of even "stable" comorbidities may affect surgical outcomes and perioperative management of these patients.

Special attention should be directed to conditions such as preexisting cardiovascular disease, particularly systemic hypertension (HTN), which may predispose the patients to hematoma formation. Preoperatively, HTN should be well controlled, and it may be prudent to either decrease the concentration of epinephrine in local anesthetic mixture, or to avoid epinephrine completely in selected patients. Evaluation of the patient's cardiac status should follow the American College of Cardiology and American Heart Association guidelines on perioperative evaluation and care for noncardiac surgery.[24] If patient's baseline functional capacity is moderate to excellent, no additional cardiac testing is required: facial cosmetic surgical procedures carry a low (<1%) risk of major cardiac complications, such as cardiac death or nonfatal myocardial infarction.[24] Preoperative and postoperative resting 12-lead electrocardiograms are not indicated in asymptomatic patients undergoing low-risk surgical procedures.[24] Likewise, routine preoperative laboratory testing before elective, low-risk ambulatory surgery is not indicated.[10,25]

Pulmonary status of patients with chronic obstructive pulmonary disease should be carefully evaluated and optimized to decrease the possibility of postoperative pulmonary complications. Cigarette smoking is associated with a 12- to 20-fold increase in risk of flap slough, and abnormal airway reactivity may provoke excessive postoperative coughing and straining, increasing the risk of postoperative bleeding.[22,23] Chronic cigarette smoking and alcohol use also cause an induction of the cytochrome P450 multienzyme system, leading to increased perioperative requirements for opioids and neuromuscular blockers, and generation of higher levels of potentially toxic metabolites of halogenated volatile anesthetic agents.[26–28]

Patients with diabetes mellitus and those with rheumatologic diseases may be particularly prone to bruising, infection, and delayed healing. The use of nonsteroidal anti-inflammatory drugs (NSAIDs), aspirin, herbal supplements such as Gingko, Echinacea, and St John's wort, and certain vitamins (eg, vitamin E) should be stopped at least 2 weeks before surgery, to avoid the risk of excessive microvascular bleeding.[22,23,29]

Healthy elderly patients can undergo office-based anesthesia safely,[10,30,31] but the anesthesiologist should be aware of pathophysiologic implications of advanced age on organ function and pharmacokinetics of anesthetic drugs. Elderly patients will require careful attention to positioning and the maintenance of intraoperative normothermia.[13]

The patients with obesity and those with the history of difficult airway should be approached with particular caution, and the anesthesiologist should be consulted early.[14] Patients with obstructive sleep apnea (OSA) should be carefully screened for suitability for same-day facial cosmetic surgery. Sleep-disordered breathing is extremely common, affecting nearly 20% of the adult population, with 7% to 8% suffering from moderate to severe OSA.[32,33] It is estimated that more than 20% of the adult surgical population suffer from OSA, which remains undiagnosed in the majority (70%) of patients.[34] When screening for the presence of OSA during a preoperative office visit, a physician may wish to use the highly sensitive and validated STOP-BANG questionnaire (Table 1).[35]

OSA adversely affects a variety of organ systems, with widespread implications for the surgical patient. The presence and severity of OSA is strongly correlated with obesity and metabolic syndrome, systemic and pulmonary HTN, congestive heart failure, arrhythmias, heart attacks, and stroke.[36–38] Patients with either known or presumed OSA should undergo outpatient surgery only if their comorbidities are optimized, if postoperative pain is going to be mild and can be predominantly managed with nonopioid analgesics, and if (for continuous positive airway pressure [CPAP] users) the patients can continue to use CPAP postoperatively.[39] For practical purposes, patients with severe OSA (ASA physical status III) should not routinely undergo office-based surgery under general anesthesia or sedation.

Intraoperatively, OSA patients demonstrate enhanced sensitivity to opioids and benzodiazepines,[40–42] which may lead to rapidly developing respiratory depression, upper airway collapse, and airway obstruction. Conscious sedation of these patients, as well as those with obesity, should be performed with extreme caution.[42,43] The OSA patients may also present with difficult airway problems, related to both difficult mask ventilation and tracheal intubation.[44–46]

Table 1	
The STOP-BANG questionnaire for screening for the risk of obstructive sleep apnea (OSA)	
Snore loudly?	**B**ody mass index >35 kg/m²?
Tired during the day?	**A**ge >50 y?
Observed cessation of breathing during sleep?	**N**eck circumference >40 cm?
Pressure (high blood pressure)?	**G**ender male?

Answering "Yes" to 3 or more questions confers a high risk of OSA. The higher the cumulative risk score, the greater the possibility of severe OSA.

A multimodal approach that minimizes narcotic medications (eg, NSAIDs, acetaminophen, cyclo-oxygenase-2–specific inhibitors) should be used perioperatively whenever feasible.[39,40] Postoperatively, the ASA recommends to extend monitoring of the OSA patients for an additional 3 hours.[47] It is best to schedule these patients earlier in the day to facilitate this, and transfer procedures to an inpatient facility should be in place should complications arise.

Patients' status should nothing by mouth on the day of surgery in accordance with the ASA Guidelines for Preoperative Fasting.[48] Clear fluid intake can be allowed for up to 2 hours before the start of surgery in otherwise healthy patients presenting for elective procedures.[48]

Premedication and Monitoring

Standard premedication with intravenous short-acting benzodiazepine (eg, midazolam) is used routinely. Antibiotic prophylaxis (eg, intravenous cefazolin) is typically administered in the majority of cases. Routine ASA monitoring is usually sufficient, even if controlled hypotension is used intraoperatively.

Patient Positioning and Prophylaxis of Thromboembolism

Ulnar neuropathies and brachial plexus injuries are most prevalent among perioperative nerve injuries, can also be observed under monitored anesthesia care (MAC),[49] but are extremely rare in cosmetic surgery. Hoefflin and colleagues[50] recorded only 1 case of peripheral neuropathy in more than 23,000 general anesthetics, perhaps reflecting the absence of risk factors for nerve damage in a healthy patient population and meticulous attention to patient positioning during office-based surgery.

Padded support (eg, lumbar area, neck) for the patient is best provided before induction of anesthesia to assure a comfortable position for the patient on the OR table for the duration of surgery, and the patient's arms and all the pressure points must be well protected intraoperatively. For MAC cases, assuring the utmost comfort of the patient on the OR table before the start of surgery will also greatly facilitate provision of anesthesia care and the patient's tolerance of long procedures. The use of forced-air warming, particularly during general anesthesia and in the elderly, facilitates maintenance of intraoperative normothermia. The patient's eyes are usually protected in the field by the surgeon.

Free access to the patient's airway is usually difficult or impossible, as the OR table is turned 90° or 180° away from the anesthesiologist. If general anesthesia is used, the anesthesiologist must thoroughly check the anesthesia circuit connections to prevent accidental disconnect under the surgical drapes, and the dedicated artificial airway must be diligently taped.

The use of the lower extremity sequential compression devices (SCDs) for prophylaxis of deep venous thrombosis (DVT) and intraoperative pulmonary embolism (PE) in anesthetized patients has become routine, and should be instituted before the induction of general anesthesia.[2,10,22]

Anesthetic Management

A wide variety of office-based cosmetic procedures can be safely and effectively performed under either local anesthesia with intravenous sedation (MAC) or general anesthesia.[3,4,50] The choice is frequently dictated by the patient's desires and the surgeon's level of comfort.[4]

Death (26%), nerve damage (22%), permanent brain damage (9%), airway injury (7%), and medication errors (7%) represent some of the most common major anesthesia-related complications, according to the ASA Closed Claims Project database containing 8954 anesthesia malpractice claims.[51] Adverse respiratory and cardiovascular incidents accounted for 17% and 13% of all claims associated with anesthesia-related sentinel events.[51] Among the respiratory incidents, difficult intubation, inadequate oxygenation or ventilation, and pulmonary aspiration were the most common,[51] and by proxy may be expected to account for the majority of patient morbidity during office-based anesthesia. In particular, inadequate oxygenation/ventilation has become a growing problem during MAC cases and administration of anesthesia in the non-OR environment.[51] Moreover, between 1997 and 2007 more than 40% of malpractice claims associated with MAC involved the patient's death or permanent brain damage.[52]

Cardiovascular incidents are not expected to be prevalent in office-based cosmetic surgery. Most cardiovascular events leading to anesthesia claims between 1990 and 2007 were related to hemorrhage/blood replacement, fluid management/electrolyte abnormalities, and stroke.[51] No major cardiovascular morbidity associated with general anesthesia was observed by Hoefflin and colleagues[50] in more than 23,000 patients who had undergone cosmetic and facial cosmetic surgery in the office-based setting.

Medication problems are relatively common, and represented 7% of anesthesia claims between 1990 and 2007.[51] These claims were fairly equally distributed between adverse drug reactions and medication errors, and most medication errors were considered preventable.[51]

Most anesthesia-related complications in ambulatory surgery are expected to be minor, with the commonly cited incidence of[53]:

- PONV 4.7%
- Shivering 2.2%
- Eye injury 0.056%
- Dental injury 0.02%
- Ulnar neuropathy 0.47%
- Sore throat 28%

Conscious sedation

Eliminating the need for general anesthesia avoids invasive airway management, removes the triggers for malignant hyperthermia and emergence phenomena, reduces the incidence of PONV, and facilitates patient discharge.[3]

The authors' experience corroborates that of others[5] that administering a successful MAC without immediate access to the patient's airway is frequently more challenging than conducting the general anesthesia. Safe management of fluctuating levels of noxious stimulation, appreciation of pharmacokinetic profile and additive and synergistic effects of administered intravenous drugs, and variability of patient responses require a high level of vigilance and skill.[51,54]

Respiratory depression resulting from either absolute or relative overdose of sedative or opioid drugs can occur at any time, and was the leading (21%) mechanism associated with inadequate oxygenation/ventilation and death/permanent brain damage in MAC malpractice claims.[52] Nearly half of these claims were judged as preventable by[52]:

1. Better monitoring, including capnography
2. Improved vigilance
3. Presence of audible monitoring alarms

MAC claims in facial cosmetic and plastic surgery are relatively common, accounting for more than 25% of all MAC claims between 1997 and 2007.[52] In the audit by Coldiron and colleagues,[8] all facial cosmetic surgical deaths were MAC related. This finding is not surprising, because during the facial procedures the visibility of the patient's airway is impaired, and capnography monitoring may become unreliable. The use of the precordial stethoscope placed over the patient's trachea to monitor breath sounds can be advantageous in such cases.

Intraoperatively, the patient care team should appreciate that MAC represents a continuum of the sedation states, which can quickly progress from a moderate level ("conscious sedation") to deeper planes whereby spontaneous ventilation

may be inadequate, and further to general anesthesia, whereby a patient becomes unresponsive and airway support will be frequently required.[55] Every planned MAC should be treated as a potential case of general anesthesia. When intravenous sedation is administered by nonanesthesiologist, at least one individual capable of establishing a patent airway and instituting positive pressure ventilation should be continually present throughout the procedure.[56]

Conducting safe and successful MAC requires the anesthesiologist to appreciate pharmacokinetic and pharmacodynamic interactions of the chosen intravenous sedating agents, as well as the role of pharmacologic antagonists for opioids and benzodiazepines.[56] A synergistic effect of the sedating agents should be kept in mind to avoid rapid onset of respiratory depression and upper airway obstruction, and the doses of the administered medications should be appropriately reduced.[43,57] The desired level(s) of sedation should be clearly defined and discussed with the surgeon preoperatively. Once these objectives are established, the choice, and the safe and rational use of intravenous sedating and hypnotic agents will largely depend on the preference and experience of the anesthesiologist.

Intravenous opioids Discussed here are:

- Remifentanil
- Alfentanil
- Midazolam
- Propofol
- Dexmedetomidine
- Ketamine

Intravenous opioids, especially those with rapid onset (alfentanil, remifentanil), may be particularly useful, as they provide intense analgesia of short duration, have a sedative effect, and possess excellent antitussive properties. One may expect almost identical peak effect time of an equipotent single bolus dose of remifentanil and alfentanil (0.9 minutes and 1.3 minutes, respectively), whereas significant delay is observed for fentanyl (3.3 minutes) and sufentanil (8.5 minutes).[58] The analgesic effect of a single bolus dose of remifentanil is 20 to 30 times higher than that of alfentanil.[59]

Remifentanil Remifentanil can be given as a bolus dose of 1 to 2 μg/kg, which is usually well tolerated by awake patients,[60] and can also be administered by infusion, which will facilitate hemodynamic stability and reduce the incidence of opioid-induced side effects.[61,62] Continuous infusions of remifentanil, 0.05 to

0.08 µg/kg/min, projected to reach a steady-state concentration of 1.3 to 2 ng/mL in 30 to 40 minutes, seem to be well tolerated by awake patients.[63–66] The anesthesiologist must keep in mind that remifentanil blood concentrations of 1.3 to 2 ng/mL are substantial, and correlate with those required to reduce minimum alveolar concentration of isoflurane by 50% and block sympathetic responses to skin incision in 50% of patients (EC_{50}) receiving target-controlled propofol anesthetic, respectively.[65,67,68]

A higher sensitivity to, and slower onset of remifentanil in the elderly should be expected, as these patients also tend to have a smaller volume of distribution and lower remifentanil clearance.[60,69] The initial loading dose of remifentanil in patients older than age 65 years should be decreased by 50% and then adjusted as required, according to the individual patient's response.[60]

Alfentanil In contrast to remifentanil, the pharmacodynamic effects of alfentanil are more variable, with the corresponding range of adequate plasma analgesic concentrations (20–60 ng/mL) for many of the awake, but sedated patients.[70,71] This concentration falls within that for adequate ventilation (EC_{50} 45–60 ng/mL) as well.[58,71] Based on the available pharmacokinetic modeling data,[70–72] a 60-ng/mL target concentration of alfentanil can probably be achieved in the majority of patients with a single alfentanil bolus dose 7 to 10 µg/kg.

Midazolam The opioids alone fail to provide sufficient levels of sedation and amnesia,[73] and their combination with intravenous benzodiazepines is usually highly desirable. Midazolam is widely used for procedural sedation, owing to its potent anxiolytic and amnestic properties, rapid effect-site equilibration, good titratability, and relatively short half-life.[73–75] However, substantial pharmacodynamic variability with regard to amnestic effect exists between the patients, and coadministration of midazolam with opioids may quickly result in oversedation, hypoventilation, apnea, or airway obstruction.[43,57,73,75] If a midazolam-remifentanil combination is used, lower doses of midazolam (1–2 mg) may be advisable[66] and careful titration is paramount. In the absence of well-defined points of titration (eg, Ramsay Sedation Scale of 2–3), administration of midazolam may result in several undesirable outcomes, such as the need for respiratory intervention that may disrupt surgery (eg, the need for airway support), slower recovery, recall despite attempted amnesia, and a risk of "atypical" reaction characterized by patient agitation necessitating a conversion to general anesthesia.[75]

Propofol Similar considerations apply to a combination of intravenous opioids with propofol. Propofol offers certain advantages over benzodiazepines, including faster onset, rapid awakening, and ease of titration.[76] The combination of opioids with propofol produces a full synergistic effect, with each drug increasing each other's sedative and analgesic properties, and this synergy is more pronounced for remifentanil than for other opioids.[58] A combination with an opioid should be expected to increase the risk of significant respiratory depression, as both the ventilatory responses to hypercapnia and hypoxemia are diminished during propofol administration.[77] If such a combination is desired, it is advisable to target an effect-site concentration lower than optimal for opioids and higher than optimal for propofol, to preserve adequate spontaneous ventilation.[58,78]

Dexmedetomidine Respiratory depression presents few issues if dexmedetomidine, a highly selective, centrally acting α2-adrenoreceptor agonist, is used for MAC.[76,79] Dexmedetomidine produces anxiolysis and sedation in a dose-dependent fashion, potentiates opioid analgesia, possesses antisialagogue, antitussive, and sympatholytic properties, and causes only minimal, if any, respiratory depression.[80–87] Thus dexmedetomidine has low likelihood for airway intervention, may decrease or eliminate supplemental oxygen requirements during laser facial cosmetic procedures, and improves patient cooperation.[75,82,88] In a retrospective study by Taghinia and colleagues[89] the use of dexmedetomidine during MAC or general anesthesia in patients undergoing face lift (rhytidectomy) resulted in reduced use of midazolam, fentanyl, and propofol, produced fewer episodes of intraoperative hypoxemia, and facilitated maintenance of intraoperative hypotension; in addition, the incidence of PONV was also reduced.

Dexmedetomidine demonstrates delayed onset of action of approximately 15 minutes, and peak concentrations are usually achieved within 1 hour following continuous intravenous infusion,[76] which make the drug poorly titratable. Nevertheless, its stable and predictable pharmacokinetic profile[79,88] makes it relatively easy to administer. A typical loading dose is 0.5 to 1.0 µg/kg bolus over 10 minutes, followed by a continuous infusion of 0.2 to 1.0 µg/kg/h, titrated to a Ramsay sedation score of 2 or greater, has been advocated.[76,84,85,88] It should be noted that the bolus doses of dexmedetomidine exceeding 1 µg/kg, especially when administered rapidly, may be associated with short periods of hypercapnia, hypoxemia, and apnea.[86]

Despite reliably producing a state of cooperative sedation, when used alone dexmedetomidine possesses little, if any, amnestic properties,[86,87] and a combination with small doses of midazolam may be desired. Analgesic properties of dexmedetomidine are also mild, and the anesthesiologist must be prepared to supplement analgesia with short-acting opioids (eg, remifentanil, alfentanil) during the most stimulating parts of the surgical procedures.[90] Again caution is needed, as this combination may result in increased likelihood of hypoventilation, apnea, and airway compromise.[75]

The limitations of the use of dexmedetomidine for outpatient surgery come from its pharmacokinetic profile and the mechanism of action. Delayed peak effect impairs clinical efficiency, and may also lead to prolonged stay in the recovery room.[75] The potent sympatholytic effect of dexmedetomidine may lead to intraoperative bradycardia and hypotension, which may persist during the recovery period; bradycardia may be further enhanced by the addition of remifentanil.[75,76,82,83]

Ketamine A combination of dexmedetomidine and ketamine may be particularly beneficial.[75] Ketamine causes sympathetic stimulation, counteracting the sympathetic depressant effects of dexmedetomidine; provides reliable and rapid amnesia; does not cause respiratory depression; and possesses analgesic properties.[75] The antisialagogue effect of dexmedetomidine offsets the ketamine-induced hypersalivation; further decrease in secretions can be enhanced by pretreatment with glycopyrrolate, which, in turn, may also counteract dexmedetomidine-induced bradycardia.[75,76] A ketamine bolus dose of 0.5 mg/kg can be recommended to induce a dissociative state of consciousness, and maintenance with a low-dose continuous infusion 3 to 10 µg/kg/min (target concentration 50–100 ng/mL)[91] should facilitate additional analgesia and the state of a light hypnosis.[75,92] Although not vigorously investigated, a combination of ketamine and propofol, popularized by Friedberg,[29] is claimed to be highly effective, allowing avoidance of the use of intraoperative opioids.

Despite its excellent safety profile, at deeper levels of sedation ketamine can still cause airway obstruction, laryngospasm, and pulmonary aspiration, especially in combination with other sedating agents.[56] Furthermore, because of the induced dissociative state, assessment of the degree of sedation with ketamine may be difficult: the patient's eyes may remain open and the eye movements may be preserved even in a state of deep sedation or general anesthesia.[56]

Successful conscious sedation The key to success of the MAC-based facial cosmetic surgery remains adequate local and regional anesthesia performed by the surgeon. The anesthesiologist and the surgeon should be thoroughly familiar with the safe total dose of a local anesthetic that can be administered to the patient. The anesthesiologist should also be made aware of the use of the local anesthetic-epinephrine mixture by the surgeon to closely observe (and treat, where appropriate) the ensuing hemodynamic responses of the patient. These responses may be exaggerated in older patients and those with coexisting cardiovascular disease, requiring prompt treatment.

Burn injuries resulting from on-patient operating room fires, particularly during head and neck surgery, have accounted for 20 MAC malpractice claims (17%) between 1997 and 2007.[52] All these burns were triggered by the use of electrocautery (diathermy), in the presence of supplemental oxygen administration to the patient, and the use of alcohol-containing prep solution and surgical drapes in the field.[52] The possibility of burn injuries during facial cosmetic surgery is reduced with general anesthesia, whereby the oxygen delivery system (eg, endotracheal tube [ETT] or laryngeal mask airway [LMA]) is usually sealed to the atmosphere. The use of the ETT or LMA is recommended for MAC with moderate to deep sedation, which require oxygen supplementation, and/or in oxygen-dependent patients who undergo surgery of the head, neck, or face.[93] The prevention and management of on-patient OR fires should follow the ASA Practice Advisory.[93] **Table 2** lists some of the most important considerations.

General anesthesia
Compared with MAC, general anesthesia[4,49]:

- Provides amnesia
- Protects the patient's airway
- Assures adequate gas exchange
- Abolishes patient movement
- Avoids distraction of the surgeon

Conventional and advanced airway manage ment Careful preoperative airway assessment should be routine, with the special attention directed to the risk factors for difficult and/or impossible mask ventilation, and their association with difficult tracheal intubation.[44–46] Previous cosmetic procedures, such as chin implant, may mask preexisting retrognathia, leading to unanticipated difficult direct laryngoscopy and intubation.[94] It is not uncommon for patients to present with extensive (and expensive) cosmetic dental work. If tracheal intubation is planned, it is the

Table 2
Prevention and management of on-patient fires in the operating room (OR)

Prevention of OR On-Patient Fires	Management of OR On-Patient Fires
Awareness and avoidance of the fire triad (oxidizer, fuel, and ignition source)	Stop the procedure and call for help
Collaboration between the members of OR team	Stop the flow of O_2 and other gases
Presence of predetermined management plan	Remove drapes and all burning/flammable material from the patient
OR fire drills	Extinguish fire with saline, water, or smothering. If unsuccessful, use CO_2 fire extinguisher
Avoid O_2 supplementation if deep levels of sedation are not planned/required	If fire persists, evacuate the patient if feasible, activate fire alarm, contain fire by closing the OR doors, turn off the medical gas supply to OR
Reduction of nasal O_2 insufflation to below 3 L/min	Assess the patient's injury and potential airway injury for smoke inhalation
Use nasopharyngeal instead of nasal O_2 insufflation to decrease O_2 concentration in the field	Administer treatment, as appropriate
Open and loose arrangement of surgical drapes around the patient's face and neck	—
Scavenging O_2 under the drapes (suction)	—
Adequate time warning to the anesthesiologist to stop/reduce O_2 before the ignition source (electrocautery, laser) is activated	—

Adapted from Refs.[52,93,165–167]

senior author's preference to eliminate the risk of dental damage by avoiding direct laryngoscopy and using alternative asleep intubation techniques, such as light-guided or flexible fiberoptic intubation.

Although tracheal intubation is probably performed most frequently,[10,50] in the absence of contraindications the use of the flexible laryngeal mask airway (FLMA; LMA North America, Inc, San Diego, CA, USA) should be given full consideration, and represents the authors' first choice. The use of the FLMA in head and neck surgery is associated with adequate airway protection, improved hemodynamic stability, superior maintenance of a stable plane of anesthesia and control of hypotension, improved quality of the surgical field, reduced usage of anesthetic drugs, shortened operative time, and faster and smoother emergence from anesthesia.[95–100] Furthermore, the use of the LMA does not require administration of NMB, facilitates the resumption of spontaneous ventilation, and is associated with decreased likelihood of the airway reflex stimulation.

When used appropriately in selected patients, absence of immediate access to the patient's airway should not be considered a deviation from the standard of care of the use of LMA in the modern era.[101] Although both spontaneous and controlled ventilation through the FLMA can be successfully performed intraoperatively, the authors usually opt for the latter (pressure control or pressure support ventilation mode), to preserve normocapnia.

The standard LMA insertion technique must be meticulously observed, and the FLMA oropharyngeal leak (OPL) pressure with the adjustable pressure-limiting valve closed on the anesthesia machine should be noted.[102] The epigastric area should be auscultated to confirm absence of gastric insufflation with positive pressure ventilation, best administered in a pressure-controlled mode at a level below the OPL pressure. Adequacy of the FLMA positioning and effectiveness of controlled ventilation should be continuously monitored intraoperatively by observing the expired tidal volume (V_t), pulse oximetry and end-tidal CO_2 ($Etco_2$) values, $Etco_2$ wave form, total leak fraction, and total compliance, and by visually assessing the flow-volume and pressure-volume loops, if available.[103] Sudden changes, such as increased leak fraction, decreased total compliance, and (depending on the mode of ventilation used) either decreased V_t or increased peak inspiratory pressure, will represent early signs of the lighter planes of anesthesia. With use of the LMA, these changes typically precede the patient's hemodynamic and motor responses, thereby facilitating hypnotic monitoring and allowing for prompt deepening of anesthesia.[103]

Anesthesia induction and maintenance Standard intravenous induction with propofol is used most often, although there is little evidence to support propofol's beneficial antiemetic effect if TIVA is not used intraoperatively.[104,105] Occasional patients may require inhalation induction because of severe needlephobia. The application of EMLA cream (a mixture of 2.5% prilocaine and 2.5% lidocaine) before the intravenous placement may be tried in these patients.

Inhalational anesthesia is probably used more commonly for maintenance of anesthesia, likely because of the ease of titratability of the inhalational agents to the patient's hemodynamic responses.[10,22,50] Sevoflurane may be preferred for the outpatient surgery, as it improves the quality of postoperative patient recovery, shortens the discharge time, is associated with reduced incidence of coughing and postoperative agitation in comparison with desflurane,[106,107] and produces less somnolence and PONV in comparison with isoflurane.[107,108] The use of nitrous oxide should be discouraged: it may provoke severe PONV, and may lead to the higher incidence of wound infection, pneumonia, atelectasis, or any other pulmonary complications.[109]

TIVA with propofol and an opioid represents the authors' anesthetic technique of choice. Most prospective studies demonstrate that, compared with inhalational and balanced inhalational techniques, TIVA is associated with superior intraoperative hemodynamic stability, quicker recovery times, faster return of cognitive function, decreased incidence of PONV, and improved patient satisfaction.[107,108,110–117]

The full synergistic effect of propofol with rapidly acting opioids, such as remifentanil or alfentanil, allows quick titration of anesthetic to the desired clinical effect.[110,112,113,118,119] Remifentanil has been shown to be superior to both fentanyl[120] and alfentanil[108,110,112,121] in promoting intraoperative hemodynamic stability, improving respiratory and general patient recovery, and facilitating patients' discharge after outpatient surgery.[108,122–125] Remifentanil can be considered a nearly ideal opioid for office-based procedures, characterized by low postoperative pain scores.[60,75]

The typical induction doses are remifentanil intravenous bolus 0.5 to 2 µg/kg and propofol intravenous bolus 1 to 2 mg/kg, followed by continuous maintenance infusions of propofol 80 to 200 µg/kg/min and remifentanil 0.1 to 0.5 µg/kg/min.[58,110,113,120,121] Commonly used doses of alfentanil are intravenous induction bolus 20 to 30 µg/kg, followed by continuous maintenance infusion 0.25 to 1 µg/kg/min.[108,110,121,126]

Postoperative pain associated with facial cosmetic surgery is low, and large doses of fentanyl or highly potent opioids, such as sufentanil, are unnecessary. In the senior author's experience, a total intraoperative dose of fentanyl can be safely limited to 1 to 2 µg/kg in most patients, especially when remifentanil is used intraoperatively.

Controlled hypotension Maintenance of moderately controlled hypotension (systolic blood pressure <100 mm Hg; mean arterial pressure 60–70 mm Hg) is essential for maintaining optimal operating conditions. A variety of pharmacologic approaches can be used, but in the authors' experience remifentanil seems to be particularly effective because of its superior potency and titratability. Maintenance of induced hypotension with remifentanil during facial cosmetic surgery rarely requires additional pharmacologic supplementation. The incidence of rebound hypertension and tachycardia also appears to be low, and prophylactic administration of labetalol intravenous bolus 0.1 to 0.3 mg/kg at the end of surgery is usually effective in patients with preexisting cardiovascular disease.[103]

Esmolol Intraoperative administration of esmolol 0.5 to 1 mg/kg intravenous bolus, followed by continuous intravenous infusion of 100 to 300 µg/kg/min, titrated to the desired hemodynamic end point[127,128] represents another effective therapeutic option. The potentiation of the effects of opioids and anesthetic agents by esmolol[129–131]:

- Further facilitates emergence from anesthesia
- Decreases postoperative opioid analgesic requirements
- May provide an effective alternative for fast-tracking patients for discharge after outpatient surgery[132–134]

PONV Shortening of the discharge time can be further improved by aggressive prevention of PONV, usually with an intravenous serotonin (5-HT$_3$) antagonist (eg, ondansetron 4–8 mg). A combination of a 5-HT$_3$ receptor blocker with intravenous dexamethasone (8–10 mg) appears to be safe and highly effective,[135,136] and may lead to improved patient outcome.[135] Intravenous dexamethasone is administered routinely during facial cosmetic surgery. Multimodal PONV prophylaxis (eg, the addition of transdermal scopolamine patch) is warranted in high-risk patients.[135,137] A recent prospective multicenter trial by Apfel and colleagues[137] has identified independent predictive factors for PONV in the postanesthesia care unit (PACU), such as female gender, age younger than 50 years, history of PONV, higher doses of intraoperative and postoperative opioids, duration of surgery longer than 1 hour, and a laparoscopic surgical approach.

At present, even with adequate antiemetic prophylaxis, the incidence of severe PONV after facial cosmetic surgery performed under balanced inhalational anesthesia does not appear to be different from that in the general patient population after ambulatory surgery: less than 5%[50,138] versus 3.8%,[137] respectively. PONV can be further reduced with TIVA, whereby the emetogenic effect of inhalational anesthetics is avoided.[135]

Emergence from anesthesia A smooth, rapid emergence with full return of the patient's protective airway reflexes is required after facial cosmetic surgery to avoid airway support and instrumentation, which may negatively affect the surgical result. Avoidance of bucking and coughing, and accompanying hypertensive responses, on emergence is essential for preventing microvascular bleeding and hematoma formation, especially after procedures such as rhinoplasty and rhytidectomy.[10,21,50,139,140]

If general endotracheal anesthesia has been used, deeper stages of anesthesia are required until the very end of the procedure to blunt the patient's laryngotracheal responses. The use of the FLMA in lieu of the ETT will facilitate smooth patient awakening and allow for safe reduction of the level of anesthesia toward the end of the surgery. Maintaining a very low-dose remifentanil intravenous infusion (eg, 0.02 µg/kg/min) until the patient is fully awakened and the FLMA is removed may be beneficial, particularly if the total intraoperative dose of intravenous fentanyl has been significantly reduced. In the senior author's experience this virtually eliminates the emergence-related events, such as patient agitation, coughing, uncontrolled head movements, and postextubation laryngospasm, even if the LMA is used.

If endotracheal intubation has been performed, smooth emergence may constitute a particularly challenging task. Extubating the patient's trachea at a deep plane of anesthesia is problematic in facial cosmetic surgery because of the increased risk of postextubation laryngospasm and overall increased need for airway support and protection required on the part of the anesthesiologist. The Bailey maneuver[141] constitutes a viable option and involves, in steps, insertion of the LMA behind the existing ETT with the patient still anesthetized,

removal of the ETT, and administration of the ventilatory support through the LMA until the patient resumes spontaneous ventilation and awakens from anesthesia. The pharmacologic approach relies on a low-dose remifentanil infusion to blunt the tracheal responses and promote smooth extubation. Remifentanil provides a predictable, rapid, and almost simultaneous recovery of consciousness and protective airway reflexes, while also blunting sympathetic responses associated with extubation.[142,143] Current data indicate that EC_{95} of effect-site concentration of remifentanil for blunting tracheal reflexes after balanced desflurane and sevoflurane anesthesia is in the range of 2.3 to 2.9 ng/mL (corresponding manual infusion rate 0.08–1.0 µg/kg/min),[144,145] higher than that observed with TIVA (target concentration 2.1 ng/mL; corresponding manual infusion rate 0.07 µg/kg/min).[146] The authors' experience corroborates that of others that lower blood target concentrations of remifentanil (1.5–2.0 ng/mL; corresponding manual infusion rate 0.05–0.06 µg/kg/min)[143,147–149] may be equally effective, especially if TIVA has been used.

Immediate postanesthesia recovery period
Patients should be observed closely for postoperative airway complications. Postoperative laryngospasm may quickly lead to the development of acute negative-pressure pulmonary edema (NPPE), which has been described after septorhinoplasty.[150] Spontaneous inspiratory efforts against the closed glottis and an obstructed upper airway generate marked negative intrapleural and transpulmonary pressures, greatly increasing venous return and pulmonary blood flow, which leads to rapid development of capillary leak and transudation of fluid into the alveolar space.[150] The fluid becomes trapped inside the lungs owing to a combination of the effects of hypoxic pulmonary vasoconstriction, an afterload increase due to massive sympathetic discharge, and depressed myocardial contractility caused by hypoxemia.[150,151] When the patient expires against a closed glottis, a Valsalva maneuver generates high auto–positive end-expiratory pressure (PEEP), preventing fluid from leaving the capillaries and entering the alveoli.[150] However, when the laryngospasm or upper airway obstruction are relieved naturally or by tracheal intubation, a rapid drop in airway pressures occurs, with prompt transudation of fluid into the alveoli, severe acute pulmonary edema, and production of pink frothy secretions.[150,151]

Postoperative laryngospasm and NPPE are infrequent events, occurring in approximately 0.3% and 0.09% of general surgical population, respectively.[150–152] Treatment is supportive, and consists of reestablishment of airway patency, oxygen supplementation, ventilatory support (CPAP, or tracheal intubation with positive pressure ventilation and PEEP), management of fluid shifts, and maintenance of normal intravascular volume.[150–152]

Postoperative control of blood pressure to prevent hematoma formation is important, particularly after rhytidectomy, whereby it can occur in up to 15% of cases.[23,140,153] Adequate analgesia and PONV prophylaxis should be provided, intravenous bolus doses of labetalol, 0.1 to 0.2 mg/kg should be administered, and the patient's head should be elevated to promote venous drainage.

Postoperative pain associated with facial cosmetic surgery is usually low, and intermittent intravenous bolus doses of fentanyl, in combination with standard oral analgesics, are usually sufficient for pain control and fast-tracking patients for discharge. Remifentanil-induced hyperalgesia has not been an issue in the authors' experience, possibly because of the relatively low rates of intravenous infusion of remifentanil typically required intraoperatively. Should acute opioid tolerance be suspected, adequate doses of fentanyl and/or long-acting opioid analgesics (eg, morphine) can be effectively and safely administered.[118]

Postoperative shivering is rare,[50] especially if TIVA has been used and normothermia has been maintained intraoperatively. Shivering can be effectively controlled with intravenous meperidine 12.5 to 25 mg,[135,154] and the addition of oral clonidine (5 μg/kg) as part of premedication has also been advocated.[29,50,154]

Postdischarge nausea and vomiting (PDNV) may occur after the patient has left the hospital, and affects more than 35% of ambulatory surgery patients.[137] The lower incidence of PONV associated with TIVA appears to be limited to the early postoperative period only.[135,137] In a large prospective multicenter trial, Apfel and colleagues[137] identified 5 independent predictive factors for PDNV after ambulatory surgery: female gender, age younger than 50 years, a history of nausea or vomiting after previous anesthesia, and opioid administration or nausea in the PACU. The main difference between the risk factors for PONV and PDNV was that patients who experienced nausea in the PACU had a 3-fold increased risk for PDNV.[137]

The patient's risk for PDNV increases progressively from approximately 10% with no risk factors, to 20% with 1 risk factor, and to 80% if all 5 risk factors are present, highlighting the need for multimodal long-acting PDNV prophylaxis with such antiemetics as dexamethasone, aprepitant (NK1 receptor antagonist), palonosetron (5-HT$_3$ antagonist), and transdermal scopolamine, either alone or in combination.[137]

The essential perioperative anesthetic considerations and requirements are summarized in **Box 2**.

Procedure-Related Anesthesia Safety Considerations

Septorhinoplasty

The risk of laryngospasm or intraoperative coughing caused by aspiration of blood and secretions is increased under MAC.[50] Under general anesthesia, the properly placed FLMA provides adequate airway protection.[95–97,100]

A rare postoperative complication consisting of concomitant paralysis of the hypoglossal and the recurrent laryngeal branch of the vagus nerve

---

Box 2
Perioperative risk reduction: essential anesthesia-related considerations

- Proper patient selection and preparation
- Routine prophylaxis of DVT and PE (use of SCDs)
- Special attention to MAC cases, especially those requiring deep sedation
- Preference for rapidly titratable drugs
- Quiet, clear surgical field: maintenance of controlled hypotension
- Absence of patient movement
- Preference for TIVA
- Avoidance of nitrous oxide
- Preference for FLMA use, whenever feasible
- Smooth, nonstimulating emergence from anesthesia
- Rapid awakening and return of protective airway reflexes
- Aggressive prevention of PONV and PDNV
- Fast-tracking patients for discharge
- Minimizing the dose of intraoperative and postoperative opioids
- Prevention of rebound hypertension
- Familiarity with procedure-specific requirements and complications

Abbreviations: DVT, deep venous thrombosis; FLMA, flexible laryngeal mask airway; MAC, monitored anesthesia care; PDNV, postdischarge nausea and vomiting; PE, pulmonary embolism; PONV, postoperative nausea and vomiting; SCD, sequential compression device; TIVA, total intravenous anesthesia.

(Tapia syndrome) has been frequently associated with general endotracheal anesthesia for septorhinoplasty, possibly resulting from excessive pressure of the throat pack in the hypopharynx.[155] There are also anecdotal reports of postoperative skull-base defects and tension pneumocephalus, which represents a medical emergency; this complication is usually a result of a poor surgical technique.[156]

Rhytidectomy

Endotracheal intubation can be commonly requested by the surgeon for these patients, because of a perceived ability to achieve a better cosmetic result by tightening the upper neck skin than when the FLMA is used (the inflated FLMA cuff sometimes provides a slight bulge around the laryngeal prominence, and may distort the neck anatomy).

Monitoring the facial-nerve twitches during a local anesthetic injection in the facial-nerve planes is desirable, to reduce the possibility of direct trauma to and paralysis of the facial nerve. The anesthesiologist must assure that the NMB has dissipated by the time the injection is performed by the surgeon. Succinylcholine can be administered for tracheal intubation, but its use in conjunction with the inhalational anesthetics may provoke malignant hyperthermia in susceptible patients. A combination of intravenous remifentanil 2 µg/kg, propofol 2 mg/kg, and lidocaine 1.5 mg/kg, and only half of an intubating dose of rocuronium (0.3 mg/kg) will achieve intubating conditions similar to those from administration of intravenous succinylcholine 1.5 mg/kg.[157] Coadministration of intravenous remifentanil bolus 3 to 4 mg/kg (or alfentanil 40–60 mg/kg) given over 90 seconds, and propofol intravenous bolus 2 to 2.5 mg/kg, will provide excellent intubating conditions without the need for NMB in the majority of patients.[158–160]

As already mentioned, aggressive control of postoperative hypertension, PONV, and PDNV is essential in preventing the formation of postoperative hematoma. Limiting intravenous fluids and bladder distension during this lengthy operation will also help in reducing postoperative patient discomfort, agitation, and hypertensive responses.

DVT and associated PE constitute some of the most feared complications of prolonged facial cosmetic surgery such as rhytidectomy. It constitutes the greatest cause of mortality after ambulatory surgery,[161] although fortunately the incidence of these complications after rhytidectomy is low. In a retrospective study of almost 10,000 rhytidectomy cases by Reinisch and colleagues,[162] the incidence of DVT was 0.35% and that of PE 0.14%, with only 1 patient death reported. Prophylaxis plays a critical role, especially under general anesthesia, whereby routine use of SCDs is strongly advisable.[22,162] Postoperatively, the emphasis should be on early ambulation and adequate pain management.[161]

Blepharoplasty

Blepharoplasty was among the top 5 cosmetic surgical procedures performed in 2011.[1] Most cases can be performed under local anesthesia with or without sedation.[50] Injection of local anesthetic into the lower eyelids may cause particular patient discomfort,[163] and may require deeper planes of intravenous sedation. The possibility of complications such as intravascular injection and damage to the globe is real,[50,163,164] and general anesthesia should be considered on an individual basis to mitigate the patient's inadvertent movement intraoperatively.

SUMMARY

As the number of cosmetic surgical procedures performed in the United States continues to grow rapidly, so does the demand for skilled anesthesia care. Although office-based anesthesia for facial cosmetic surgery remains remarkably safe, no anesthesia or sedation performed outside the OR should be considered minor.[5] Proper organization, preparation, and patient selection, close collaboration with the surgeon, and expert and effective anesthesia care will increase patient safety, and improve perioperative outcomes and patient satisfaction.

REFERENCES

1. The American Society for Aesthetic Plastic Surgery's (ASAPS) statistics: complete charts. 2011. Available at: http://www.surgery.org/media/statistics. Accessed April 1, 2013.
2. Keyes GR, Singer R, Iverson RE, et al. Mortality in outpatient surgery. Plast Reconstr Surg 2008;12: 245–50.
3. Blake DR. Office-based anesthesia: dispelling common myths. Aesthet Surg J 2008;28:564–70.
4. Bitar G, Mullis W, Jacobs W, et al. Safety and efficacy of office-based surgery with monitored anesthesia care/sedation in 4778 consecutive plastic surgery procedures. Plast Reconstr Surg 2003; 111:150–6.
5. Melloni C. Anesthesia and sedation outside the operating room: how to prevent risk and maintain good quality. Curr Opin Anaesthesiol 2007;20: 513–9.
6. Byrd HS, Barton FE, Orenstein HH, et al. Safety and efficacy in an accredited outpatient plastic

surgery facility: a review of 5316 consecutive cases. Plast Reconstr Surg 2003;112:636–41.

7. Hancox JG, Venkat AP, Coldiron B, et al. The safety of office-based surgery: review of recent literature from several disciplines. Arch Dermatol 2004;140: 1379–82.

8. Coldiron B, Shreve E, Balkrishnan R. Patient injuries from surgical procedures performed in medical offices: three years of Florida data. Dermatol Surg 2004;30:1435–43.

9. Guidelines for Ambulatory Anesthesia and Surgery Committee of Origin: Ambulatory Surgical Care (Approved by the ASA House of Delegates on October 15, 2003, and last amended on October 22, 2008); Guidelines for Office-Based Anesthesia Committee of Origin: Ambulatory Surgical Care (Approved by the ASA House of Delegates on October 13, 1999, and last affirmed on October 21, 2009); Standards for Basic Anesthetic Monitoring Committee of Origin: Standards and Practice Parameters (Approved by the ASA House of Delegates on October 21, 1986, and last amended on October 20, 2010 with an effective date of July 1, 2011); Standards for Postanesthesia Care Committee of Origin: Standards and Practice Parameters (Approved by the ASA House of Delegates on October 27, 2004, and last amended on October 21, 2009) Guidelines. Available at: http://www. asahq.org/For-Members/Standards-Guidelines-and-Statements.aspx. Accessed June 1, 2013.

10. Caloss R, Lard MD. Anesthesia for office-based facial cosmetic surgery. Atlas Oral Maxillofac Surg Clin North Am 2004;12:163–77.

11. Eichhorn V, Henzler D, Murphy MF. Standardizing care and monitoring for anesthesia or procedural sedation delivered outside the operating room. Curr Opin Anaesthesiol 2010;23:494–9.

12. Evron S, Ezri T. Organizational prerequisites for anesthesia outside the operating room. Curr Opin Anaesthesiol 2009;22:514–8.

13. Ellsworth WA, Basu CB, Iverson RE. Perioperative considerations for patient safety during cosmetic surgery—preventing complications. Can J Plast Surg 2009;17:9–16.

14. Kurrek MM, Twersky RS. Office-based anesthesia. Can J Anaesth 2010;57:256–72.

15. Merrill D. Management of outcomes in the ambulatory surgery center: the role of standard work and evidence-based medicine. Curr Opin Anaesthesiol 2008;21:743–7.

16. de Vries EN, Prins HA, Crolla RM, et al. Effect of a comprehensive surgical safety system on patient outcomes. N Engl J Med 2010;363:1928–37.

17. de Vries EN, Eikens-Jansen MP, Hamersma AM, et al. Prevention of surgical malpractice claims by use of a surgical safety checklist. Ann Surg 2011; 253:624–8.

18. Safety checklist for office-based surgery, developed by The Institute for Safety in Office-Based Surgery (ISOBS). Available at: http://www.apsf.org/newsletters/html/2011/spring/images/checklistlg.jpg. Accessed April 1, 2013.

19. Rosenberg NM, Urman RD, Gallagher S, et al. Effect of an office-based surgical safety system on patient outcomes. Eplasty 2012;12:e59.

20. Metzner J, Posner KL, Domino KB. The risk and safety of anesthesia at remote locations: the US closed claims analysis. Curr Opin Anaesthesiol 2009;22:502–8.

21. Taub PJ, Bashey S, Hausman LM. Anesthesia for cosmetic surgery. Plast Reconstr Surg 2010;125: 1e–7e.

22. Prendiville S, Weiser S. Management of anesthesia and facility in facelift surgery. Facial Plast Surg Clin North Am 2009;17:531–8.

23. Clevens RA. Avoiding patient dissatisfaction and complications in facelift surgery. Facial Plast Surg Clin North Am 2009;17:515–30.

24. Fleisher LA, Beckman JA, Brown KA, et al. ACC/AHA 2007 guidelines on perioperative cardiovascular evaluation and care for noncardiac surgery: a report of the American College of Cardiology/American Heart Association Task Force on Practice Guidelines (Writing Committee to Revise the 2002 Guidelines on Perioperative Cardiovascular Evaluation for Noncardiac Surgery) developed in collaboration with the American Society of Echocardiography, American Society of Nuclear Cardiology, Heart Rhythm Society, Society of Cardiovascular Anesthesiologists, Society for Cardiovascular Angiography and Interventions, Society for Vascular Medicine and Biology, and Society for Vascular Surgery. J Am Coll Cardiol 2007;50:e159–241.

25. Benarroch-Gampel J, Sheffield KM, Duncan CB, et al. Preoperative laboratory testing in patients undergoing elective, low-risk ambulatory surgery. Ann Surg 2012;256:518–28.

26. Lieber CS. Ethanol metabolism, cirrhosis and alcoholism. Clin Chim Acta 1997;257:59–84.

27. McKillop IH, Schrum LW. Alcohol and liver cancer. Alcohol 2005;35:195–203.

28. Sweeney BP, Bromilow J. Liver enzyme induction and inhibition: implications for anaesthesia. Anaesthesia 2006;61:159–77.

29. Friedberg BL. Propofol-ketamine technique: dissociative anesthesia for office surgery (a 5-year review of 1264 cases). Aesthetic Plast Surg 1999; 23:70–5.

30. Fleisher LA, Pasternak LR, Herbert R, et al. Inpatient hospital admission and death after outpatient surgery in elderly patients: importance of patient and system characteristics and location of care. Arch Surg 2004;139:67–72.

31. Bettelli G. High risk patients in day surgery. Minerva Anestesiol 2009;75:259–68.

32. Isono S. Obstructive sleep apnea of obese adults: pathophysiology and perioperative airway management. Anesthesiology 2009;110:908–21.

33. Lopez PP, Stefan B, Schulman CI, et al. Prevalence of sleep apnea in morbidly obese patients who presented for weight loss surgery evaluation: more evidence for routine screening for obstructive sleep apnea before weight loss surgery. Am Surg 2008; 74:834–8.

34. Finkel KJ, Searleman AC, Tymkew H, et al. Prevalence of undiagnosed obstructive sleep apnea among adult surgical patients in an academic medical center. Sleep Med 2009;10:753–8.

35. Chung F, Yegneswaran B, Liao P, et al. STOP questionnaire: a tool to screen patients for obstructive sleep apnea. Anesthesiology 2008;108:812–21.

36. Adesanya AO, Lee W, Greilich NB, et al. Perioperative management of obstructive sleep apnea. Chest 2010;138:1489–98.

37. Somers VK, White DP, Amin R, et al. Sleep apnea and cardiovascular disease: an American Heart Association/American College Of Cardiology Foundation Scientific Statement from the American Heart Association Council for High Blood Pressure Research Professional Education Committee, Council on Clinical Cardiology, Stroke Council, and Council On Cardiovascular Nursing. Circulation 2008;118:1080–111.

38. Woodson BT, Franco R. Physiology of sleep disordered breathing. Otolaryngol Clin North Am 2007; 40:691–711.

39. Joshi GP, Ankichetty SP, Gan TJ, et al. Society for Ambulatory Anesthesia consensus statement on preoperative selection of adult patients with obstructive sleep apnea scheduled for ambulatory surgery. Anesth Analg 2012;115:1060–8.

40. Chung F, Elsaid H. Screening for obstructive sleep apnea before surgery: why is it important? Curr Opin Anaesthesiol 2009;22:405–11.

41. Chung SA, Yuan H, Chung F. A systemic review of obstructive sleep apnea and its implications for anesthesiologists. Anesth Analg 2008;107: 1543–63.

42. Hillman DR, Platt PR, Eastwood PR. Anesthesia, sleep, and upper airway collapsibility. Anesthesiol Clin 2010;28:443–55.

43. Drummond GB. Comparison of sedation with midazolam and ketamine: effects on airway muscle activity. Br J Anaesth 1996;76:663–7.

44. Langeron O, Masso E, Huraux C, et al. Prediction of difficult mask ventilation. Anesthesiology 2000; 92:1229–36.

45. Kheterpal S, Han R, Tremper KK, et al. Incidence and predictors of difficult and impossible mask ventilation. Anesthesiology 2006;105:885–91.

46. Kheterpal S, Martin L, Shanks AM, et al. Prediction and outcomes of impossible mask ventilation: a review of 50,000 anesthetics. Anesthesiology 2009; 110:891–7.

47. Gross JB, Bachenberg KL, Benumof JL, et al. Practice guidelines for the perioperative management of patients with obstructive sleep apnea: a report by the American Society of Anesthesiologists Task Force on Perioperative Management of patients with obstructive sleep apnea. Anesthesiology 2006;104:1081–93.

48. American Society of Anesthesiologists Committee. Practice guidelines for preoperative fasting and the use of pharmacologic agents to reduce the risk of pulmonary aspiration: application to healthy patients undergoing elective procedures: an updated report by the American Society of Anesthesiologists Committee on Standards and Practice Parameters. Anesthesiology 2011;114:495–511.

49. Cheney FW, Domino KB, Caplan RA, et al. Nerve injury associated with anesthesia: a closed claims analysis. Anesthesiology 1999;90:1062–9.

50. Hoefflin SM, Bornstein JB, Gordon M. General anesthesia in an office-based plastic surgical facility: a report on more than 23,000 consecutive office-based procedures under general anesthesia with no significant anesthetic complications. Plast Reconstr Surg 2001;107:243–51.

51. Metzner J, Posner KL, Lam MS, et al. Closed claims' analysis. Best Pract Res Clin Anaesthesiol 2011;25:263–76.

52. Bhananker SM, Posner KL, Cheney FW, et al. Injury and liability associated with monitored anesthesia care: a closed claims analysis. Anesthesiology 2006;104:228–34.

53. Waddle J, Coleman J. General anesthesia in an office-based plastic surgical facility: a report on more than 23,000 consecutive office-based procedures under general anesthesia with no significant anesthetic complications by Steven M. Hoefflin, M.D., John B. Bornstein, M.D., Martin Gordon, M.D [discussion]. Plast Reconstr Surg 2001;107: 256–7.

54. Hug CC. MAC should stand for maximum anesthesia caution, not minimal anesthesiology care. Anesthesiology 2006;104:221–3.

55. Continuum of Depth of Sedation: Definition of General Anesthesia and Levels of Sedation/Analgesia* Committee of Origin: Quality Management and Departmental Administration (Approved by the ASA House of Delegates on October 13, 1999, and amended on October 21, 2009). Available at: http://www.asahq.org/For-Members/Standards-Guidelines-and-Statements.aspx. Accessed June 1, 2013.

56. American Society of Anesthesiologists Task Force on Sedation and Analgesia by Non-Anesthesiologists. Practice guidelines for sedation and analgesia

by non-anesthesiologists. Anesthesiology 2002;96:1004–17.

57. Bailey PL, Pace NL, Ashburn MA, et al. Frequent hypoxemia and apnea after sedation with midazolam and fentanyl. Anesthesiology 1990;73:826–30.

58. Vuyk J. Clinical interpretation of pharmacokinetic and pharmacodynamic propofol-opioid interactions. Acta Anaesthesiol Belg 2001;52:445–51.

59. Glass PS, Hardman D, Kamiyama Y, et al. Preliminary pharmacokinetics and pharmacodynamics of an ultra-short-acting opioid: remifentanil (GI87084B). Anesth Analg 1993;77:1031–40.

60. Glass PS, Gan TJ, Howell S. A review of the pharmacokinetics and pharmacodynamics of remifentanil. Anesth Analg 1999;89:S7–14.

61. Ausems ME, Vuyk J, Hug CC Jr, et al. Comparison of a computer-assisted infusion versus intermittent bolus administration of alfentanil as a supplement to nitrous oxide for lower abdominal surgery. Anesthesiology 1988;68:851–61.

62. Kern SE, Stanski DR. Pharmacokinetics and pharmacodynamics of intravenously administered anesthetic drugs: concepts and lessons for drug development. Clin Pharmacol Ther 2008;84:153–7.

63. Gustorff B, Anzenhofer S, Sycha T, et al. The sunburn pain model: the stability of primary and secondary hyperalgesia over 10 hours in a crossover setting. Anesth Analg 2004;98:173–7.

64. Gustorff B, Hoechtl K, Sycha T, et al. The effects of remifentanil and gabapentin on hyperalgesia in a new extended inflammatory skin pain model in healthy volunteers. Anesth Analg 2003;98:401–7.

65. Lang E, Kapila A, Shlugman D, et al. Reduction of isoflurane minimal alveolar concentration by remifentanil. Anesthesiology 1996;85:721–8.

66. Gold MI, Watkins WD, Sung YF, et al. Remifentanil versus remifentanil/midazolam for ambulatory surgery during monitored anesthesia care. Anesthesiology 1997;87:51–7.

67. Albertin A, Casati A, Federica L, et al. The effect-site concentration of remifentanil blunting cardiovascular responses to tracheal intubation and skin incision during bispectral index-guided propofol anesthesia. Anesth Analg 2005;101:125–30.

68. Munoz HR, Cortinez LI, Ibacache ME, et al. Remifentanil requirements during propofol administration to block the somatic responses to skin incision in children and adults. Anesth Analg 2007;104:77–80.

69. Minto CF, Schnider TW, Egan TD, et al. Influence of age and gender on the pharmacokinetics and pharmacodynamics of remifentanil. I. Model development. Anesthesiology 1997;86:10–23.

70. Van den Nieuwenhuyzen MC, Engbers FH, Burm AG, et al. Target-controlled infusion of alfentanil for postoperative analgesia: a feasibility study and pharmacodynamic evaluation in the early postoperative period. Br J Anaesth 1997;78:17–23.

71. Irwin MG, Campbell RC, Lun TS, et al. Patient maintained alfentanil target-controlled infusion for analgesia during extracorporeal shock wave lithotripsy. Can J Anaesth 1996;43:919–24.

72. Glass PS, Iselin-Chaves IA, Goodman D, et al. Determination of the potency of remifentanil compared with alfentanil using ventilatory depression as the measure of opioid effect. Anesthesiology 1999;90:1556–63.

73. Avramov MN, Smith I, White PF. Interactions between midazolam and remifentanil during monitored anesthesia care. Anesthesiology 1996;85:1283–9.

74. Lai HC, Hung CJ, Tsai YS, et al. Co-administration of midazolam decreases propofol dose during anesthesia in endoscopic laryngeal microsurgery. Acta Anaesthesiol Sin 1996;34:191–6.

75. Atkins JH, Mirza N. Anesthetic considerations and surgical caveats for awake airway surgery. Anesthesiol Clin 2010;28:555–75.

76. Szumita PM, Baroletti SA, Anger KE, et al. Sedation and analgesia in the intensive care unit: evaluating the role of dexmedetomidine. Am J Health Syst Pharm 2007;64:37–44.

77. Nieuwenhuijs D, Sarton E, Teppema L, et al. Propofol for monitored anesthesia care: implications on hypoxic control of cardiorespiratory responses. Anesthesiology 2000;92:46–54.

78. Passot S, Servin F, Allary R, et al. Target-controlled versus manually-controlled infusion of propofol for direct laryngoscopy and bronchoscopy. Anesth Analg 2002;94:1212–6.

79. Maze M, Scarfini C, Cavaliere F. New agents for sedation in the intensive care unit. Crit Care Clin 2001;17:881–97.

80. Kamibayashi T, Maze M. Clinical uses of alpha2-adrenergic agonists. Anesthesiology 2000;93:1345–9.

81. Abdelmalak B, Makary L, Hoban J, et al. Dexmedetomidine as sole sedative for awake intubation in management of the critical airway. J Clin Anesth 2007;19:370–3.

82. Shukry M, Miller JA. Update on dexmedetomidine: use in nonintubated patients requiring sedation for surgical procedures. Ther Clin Risk Manag 2010;6:111–21.

83. Coursin DB, Coursin DB, Maccioli GA. Dexmedetomidine. Curr Opin Crit Care 2001;7:221–6.

84. Bergese SD, Candiotti KA, Bokesch PM, et al, AWAKE Study Group. A Phase IIIb, randomized, double-blind, placebo-controlled, multicenter study evaluating the safety and efficacy of dexmedetomidine for sedation during awake fiberoptic intubation. Am J Ther 2010;17:586–95.

85. Bergese SD, Patrick Bender S, McSweeney TD, et al. A comparative study of dexmedetomidine with midazolam and midazolam alone for sedation during elective awake fiberoptic intubation. J Clin Anesth 2010;22:35–40.

86. Ebert TJ, Hall JE, Barney JA, et al. The effects of increasing plasma concentrations of dexmedetomidine in humans. Anesthesiology 2000;93: 382–94.

87. Hall JE, Uhrich TD, Barney JA, et al. Sedative, amnestic, and analgesic properties of small-dose dexmedetomidine infusions. Anesth Analg 2000;90: 699–705.

88. Candiotti KA, Bergese SD, Bokesch PM, et al, MAC Study Group. Monitored anesthesia care with dexmedetomidine: a prospective, randomized, double-blind, multicenter trial. Anesth Analg 2010; 110:47–56.

89. Taghinia AH, Shapiro FE, Slavin SA. Dexmedetomidine in aesthetic facial surgery: improving anesthetic safety and efficacy. Plast Reconstr Surg 2008;121:269–71.

90. Busick T, Kussman M, Scheidt T, et al. Preliminary experience with dexmedetomidine for monitored anesthesia care during ENT surgical procedures. Am J Ther 2008;15:520–7.

91. Luginbühl M, Gerber A, Schnider TW, et al. Modulation of remifentanil-induced analgesia, hyperalgesia, and tolerance by small-dose ketamine in humans. Anesth Analg 2003;96:726–32.

92. Schmid RL, Sandler AN, Katz J. Use and efficacy of low-dose ketamine in the management of acute postoperative pain: a review of current techniques and outcomes. Pain 1999;82:111–25.

93. Apfelbaum JL, Caplan RA, Barker SJ, et al. Practice advisory for the prevention and management of operating room fires: an updated report by the American Society of Anesthesiologists Task Force on Operating Room Fires. Anesthesiology 2013; 118:271–90.

94. Haddow GR, Brodsky JB, Brock-Utne JG, et al. Difficult laryngoscopy masked by previous cosmetic surgery. Plast Reconstr Surg 1991;87: 1143–4.

95. Webster AC, Morley-Forster PK, Janzen V, et al. Anesthesia for intranasal surgery: a comparison between tracheal intubation and the flexible reinforced laryngeal mask airway. Anesth Analg 1999;88:421–5.

96. Atef A, Fawaz A. Comparison of laryngeal mask with endotracheal tube for anesthesia in endoscopic sinus surgery. Am J Rhinol 2008;22:653–7.

97. Ahmed MZ, Vohra A. The reinforced laryngeal mask airway (RLMA) protects the airway in patients undergoing nasal surgery - an observational study of 200 patients. Can J Anaesth 2002;49:863–6.

98. Keller C, Brimacombe J. The influence of head and neck position on oropharyngeal leak pressure and cuff position with the flexible and the standard laryngeal mask airway. Anesth Analg 1999;88: 913–6.

99. Nair I, Bailey PM. Review of uses of the laryngeal mask in ENT anaesthesia. Anaesthesia 1995;50: 898–900.

100. Kaplan A, Crosby GJ, Bhattacharyya N. Airway protection and the laryngeal mask airway in sinus and nasal surgery. Laryngoscope 2004;114:652–5.

101. Mandel JE. Laryngeal mask airways in ear, nose, and throat procedures. Anesthesiol Clin 2010;28: 469–83.

102. Keller C, Brimacombe JR, Keller K, et al. Comparison of four methods for assessing airway sealing pressure with the laryngeal mask airway in adult patients. Br J Anaesth 1999;82:286–7.

103. Nekhendzy V. Anesthesia for otologic and neurotologic surgery. In: Abdelmalak B, Doyle DJ, editors. Anesthesia for otolaryngologic surgery. London: Cambridge University Press; 2013. p. 271–95.

104. Soppitt AJ, Glass PS, Howell S, et al. The use of propofol for its antiemetic effect: a survey of clinical practice in the United States. J Clin Anesth 2000; 12:265–9.

105. Tramèr M, Moore A, McQuay H. Propofol anaesthesia and postoperative nausea and vomiting: quantitative systematic review of randomized controlled studies. Br J Anaesth 1997;78.247–55.

106. White PF, Tang J, Wender RH, et al. Desflurane versus sevoflurane for maintenance of outpatient anesthesia: the effect on early versus late recovery and perioperative coughing. Anesth Analg 2009; 109:387–93.

107. Gupta A, Stierer T, Zuckerman R, et al. Comparison of recovery profile after ambulatory anesthesia with propofol, isoflurane, sevoflurane and desflurane: a systematic review. Anesth Analg 2004;98:632–41.

108. Philip BK, Kallar SK, Bogetz MS, et al. A multicenter comparison of maintenance and recovery with sevoflurane or isoflurane for adult ambulatory anesthesia. The Sevoflurane Multicenter Ambulatory Group. Anesth Analg 1996;83:314–9.

109. Graham AM, Myles PS, Leslie K, et al. A cost-benefit analysis of the ENIGMA trial. Anesthesiology 2011;115:265–72.

110. Eberhart LH, Eberspaecher M, Wulf H, et al. Fast-track eligibility, costs and quality of recovery after intravenous anaesthesia with propofol-remifentanil versus balanced anaesthesia with isoflurane-alfentanil. Eur J Anaesthesiol 2004;21:107–14.

111. Van den Berg AA, Savva D, Honjol NM, et al. Comparison of total intravenous, balanced inhalational and combined intravenous-inhalational anaesthesia for tympanoplasty, septorhinoplasty and

adenotonsillectomy. Anaesth Intensive Care 1995; 23:574–82.

112. Loop T, Priebe HJ. Recovery after anesthesia with remifentanil combined with propofol, desflurane, or sevoflurane for otorhinolaryngeal surgery. Anesth Analg 2000;91:123–9.

113. Montes FR, Trillos JE, Rincón IE, et al. Comparison of total intravenous anesthesia and sevoflurane-fentanyl anesthesia for outpatient otorhinolaryngeal surgery. J Clin Anesth 2002;14:324–8.

114. Larsen B, Seitz A, Larsen R. Recovery of cognitive function after remifentanil-propofol anesthesia: a comparison with desflurane and sevoflurane anesthesia. Anesth Analg 2000;90:168–74.

115. Visser K, Hassink EA, Bonsel GJ, et al. Randomized controlled trial of total intravenous anesthesia with propofol versus inhalation anesthesia with isoflurane-nitrous oxide: postoperative nausea with vomiting and economic analysis. Anesthesiology 2001;95:616–26.

116. Siler JN, Horrow JC, Rosenberg H. Propofol reduces prolonged outpatient PACU stay. An analysis according to surgical procedure. Anesthesiol Rev 1994;21:129–32.

117. Tang J, Chen L, White PF, et al. Recovery profile, costs, and patient satisfaction with propofol and sevoflurane for fast-track office-based anesthesia. Anesthesiology 1999;91:253–61.

118. Mustola ST, Baer GA, Neuvonen PJ, et al. Requirements of propofol at different end-points without adjuvant and during two different steady infusions of remifentanil. Acta Anaesthesiol Scand 2005;49: 215–21.

119. Pavlin JD, Colley PS, Weymuller EA Jr, et al. Propofol versus isoflurane for endoscopic sinus surgery. Am J Otolaryngol 1999;20:96–101.

120. Twersky RS, Jamerson B, Warner DS, et al. Hemodynamics and emergence profile of remifentanil versus fentanyl prospectively compared in a large population of surgical patients. J Clin Anesth 2001;13:407–16.

121. Wuesten R, Van Aken H, Glass PS, et al. Assessment of depth of anesthesia and postoperative respiratory recovery after remifentanil- versus alfentanil-based total intravenous anesthesia in patients undergoing ear-nose-throat surgery. Anesthesiology 2001;94:211–7.

122. Wiel E, Davette M, Carpentier L, et al. Comparison of remifentanil and alfentanil during anaesthesia for patients undergoing direct laryngoscopy without intubation. Br J Anaesth 2003;91:421–3.

123. Ozkose Z, Yalcin Cok O, Tuncer B, et al. Comparison of hemodynamics, recovery profile, and early postoperative pain control and costs of remifentanil versus alfentanil-based total intravenous anesthesia (TIVA). J Clin Anesth 2002;14:161–8.

124. Alper I, Erhan E, Ugur G, et al. Remifentanil versus alfentanil in total intravenous anaesthesia for day case surgery. Eur J Anaesthesiol 2003; 20:61–4.

125. Pandazi AK, Louizos AA, Davilis DJ, et al. Inhalational anesthetic technique in microlaryngeal surgery: a comparison between sevoflurane-remifentanil and sevoflurane-alfentanil anesthesia. Ann Otol Rhinol Laryngol 2003;112:373–8.

126. Stanski DR, Shafer SL. Quantifying anesthetic drug interaction. Implications for drug dosing. Anesthesiology 1995;83:1–5.

127. Degoute CS. Controlled hypotension: a guide to drug choice. Drugs 2007;67:1053–76.

128. Yu SK, Tait G, Karkouti K, et al. The safety of perioperative esmolol: a systematic review and meta-analysis of randomized controlled trials. Anesth Analg 2011;112:267–81.

129. Miller DR, Martineau RJ, Wynands JE, et al. Bolus administration of esmolol for controlling the haemodynamic response to tracheal intubation: the Canadian Multicentre Trial. Can J Anaesth 1991; 38:849–58.

130. Menigaux C, Guignard B, Adam F, et al. Esmolol prevents movement and attenuates the BIS response to orotracheal intubation. Br J Anaesth 2002;89:857–62.

131. Oda Y, Nishikawa K, Hase I, et al. The short-acting beta1-adrenoceptor antagonists esmolol and landiolol suppress the bispectral index response to tracheal intubation during sevoflurane anesthesia. Anesth Analg 2005;100:733–7.

132. White PF, Wang B, Tang J, et al. The effect of intraoperative use of esmolol and nicardipine on recovery after ambulatory surgery. Anesth Analg 2003; 97:1633–8.

133. Coloma M, Chiu JW, White PF, et al. The use of esmolol as an alternative to remifentanil during desflurane anesthesia for fast-track outpatient gynecologic laparoscopic surgery. Anesth Analg 2001;92:352–7.

134. Smith I, Van Hemelrijck J, White PF. Efficacy of esmolol versus alfentanil as a supplement to propofol-nitrous oxide anesthesia. Anesth Analg 1991;73:540–6.

135. Kolodzie K, Apfel CC. Nausea and vomiting after office-based anesthesia. Curr Opin Anaesthesiol 2009;22:532–8.

136. Liu YH, Li MJ, Wang PC, et al. Use of dexamethasone on the prophylaxis of nausea and vomiting after tympanomastoid surgery. Laryngoscope 2001; 111:1271–4.

137. Apfel CC, Philip BK, Cakmakkaya OS, et al. Who is at risk for postdischarge nausea and vomiting after ambulatory surgery? Anesthesiology 2012;117: 475–86.

138. Steely RL, Collins DR Jr, Cohen BE, et al. Postoperative nausea and vomiting in the plastic surgery patient. Aesthetic Plast Surg 2004;28:29–32.

139. Niamtu J. Expanding hematoma in face-lift surgery: literature review, case presentations, and caveats. Dermatol Surg 2005;31:1134–44.

140. Beer GM, Goldscheider E, Weber A, et al. Prevention of acute hematoma after face-lifts. Aesthetic Plast Surg 2010;34:502–7.

141. Verghese C. Laryngeal mask airway devices: three maneuvers for any clinical situation. Available at: http://www.anesthesiologynews.com/download/3Maneuvers_ANGAM10_WM.pdf. Accessed January 4, 2013.

142. Rees L, Mason RA. Advanced upper airway obstruction in ENT surgery. Br J Anaesth CEPD Reviews 2002;2:134–8.

143. Nho JS, Lee SY, Kang JM, et al. Effects of maintaining a remifentanil infusion on the recovery profiles during emergence from anaesthesia and tracheal extubation. Br J Anaesth 2009;103:817–21.

144. Cho HB, Kim JY, Kim DH, et al. Comparison of the optimal effect-site concentrations of remifentanil for preventing cough during emergence from desflurane or sevoflurane anesthesia. J Int Med Res 2012;40:174 83.

145. Choi EM, Park WK, Choi SH, et al. Smooth emergence in men undergoing nasal surgery: the effect cito concentration of remifentanil for preventing cough after sevoflurane-balanced anesthesia. Acta Anaesthesiol Scand 2012;56:498–503.

146. Lee B, Lee JR, Na S. Targeting smooth emergence: the effect site concentration of remifentanil for preventing cough during emergence during propofol-remifentanil anaesthesia for thyroid surgery. Br J Anaesth 2009;102:775–8.

147. Jun NH, Lee JW, Song JW, et al. Optimal effect-site concentration of remifentanil for preventing cough during emergence from sevoflurane-remifentanil anesthesia. Anaesthesia 2010;65:930–5.

148. Kim H, Choi SH, Choi YS, et al. Comparison of the antitussive effect of remifentanil during recovery from propofol and sevoflurane anesthesia. Anaesthesia 2012;67:765–70.

149. Machata AM, Illievich UM, Gustorff B, et al. Remifentanil for tracheal tube tolerance: a case control study. Anaesthesia 2007;62:796–801.

150. Westreich R, Sampson I, Shaari CM, et al. Negative-pressure pulmonary edema after routine septorhinoplasty: discussion of pathophysiology, treatment, and prevention. Arch Facial Plast Surg 2006;8:8–15.

151. Chuang YC, Wang CH, Lin YS. Negative pressure pulmonary edema: report of three cases and review of the literature. Eur Arch Otorhinolaryngol 2007;264:1113–6.

152. Mamiya H, Ichinohe T, Kaneko Y. Negative pressure pulmonary edema after oral and maxillofacial surgery. Anesth Prog 2009;56:49–52.

153. Bloom JD, Immerman SB, Rosenberg DB. Face-lift complications. Facial Plast Surg 2012;28:260–72.

154. Park SM, Mangat HS, Berger K, et al. Efficacy spectrum of antishivering medications: meta-analysis of randomized controlled trials. Crit Care Med 2012;40:3070–82.

155. Lykoudis EG, Seretis K. Tapia's syndrome: an unexpected but real complication of rhinoplasty: case report and literature review. Aesthetic Plast Surg 2012;36:557–9.

156. Naraghi M, Ghazizadeh M. Tension pneumocephalus: a life-threatening complication of septoplasty and septorhinoplasty. B-ENT 2012;8:203–5.

157. Siddik-Sayyid SM, Taha SK, Kanazi GE, et al. Excellent intubating conditions with remifentanil-propofol and either low-dose rocuronium or succinylcholine. Can J Anaesth 2009;56:483–8.

158. Scheller MS, Zornow MH, Saidman LJ. Tracheal intubation without the use of muscle relaxants: a technique using propofol and varying doses of alfentanil. Anesth Analg 1992;75:788–93.

159. Erhan E, Ugur G, Alper I, et al. Tracheal intubation without muscle relaxants: remifentanil or alfentanil in combination with propofol. Eur J Anaesthesiol 2003;20:37 43.

160. Erhan E, Ugur G, Gunusen I, et al. Propofol—not thiopental or etomidate—with remifentanil provides adequate intubating conditions in the absence of neuromuscular blockade. Can J Anaesth 2003;50:108–15.

161. Shapiro FE. Anesthesia for outpatient cosmetic surgery. Curr Opin Anaesthesiol 2008;21:704–10.

162. Reinisch JF, Bresnick SD, Walker JW, et al. Deep venous thrombosis and pulmonary embolus after face lift: a study of incidence and prophylaxis. Plast Reconstr Surg 2001;107:1570–5.

163. Whipple KM, Lim LH, Korn BS, et al. Blepharoplasty complications: prevention and management. Clin Plast Surg 2013;40:213–24.

164. Oestreicher J, Mehta S. Complications of blepharoplasty: prevention and management. Plast Surg Int 2012;2012:252368.

165. Meneghetti SC, Morgan MM, Fritz J, et al. Operating room fires: optimizing safety. Plast Reconstr Surg 2007;20:1701–8.

166. Engel SJ, Patel NK, Morrison CM, et al. Operating room fires: part II. Optimizing safety. Plast Reconstr Surg 2012;130:681–9.

167. Orhan-Sungur M, Komatsu R, Sherman A, et al. Effect of nasal cannula oxygen administration on oxygen concentration at facial and adjacent landmarks. Anaesthesia 2009;64:521–6.

Complications of Patient Selection
Recognizing the Difficult Patient

Richard L. Goode, MD

KEYWORDS

- Unhappy patient • Patient selection • Facial plastic surgery candidates

KEY POINTS

- The axiom that "the surgeon makes his/her living from the patients on whom he operates while he makes his reputation from those he refuses to operate" is very true, but is hard to do.
- Patients who are easy to reject for surgical procedures include:
  - Other surgeons' complications
  - Litigious patients
  - Patients the surgeon or his or staff do not like
  - Patients with a psychiatric disorder
  - Patients with a body dysmorphic disorder
  - Patients with multiple medical comorbidities
- Patients who are difficult to evaluate for selecting for surgical procedures, include, among others:
  - Depressed patients
  - Minor deformity patients
  - Doctor shoppers
  - Patients who have had several plastic surgery procedures by others
  - Super fastidious patient
  - Family members and close friends
  - Heavy smokers
  - Chronic pain patients on daily pain medications

INTRODUCTION

The procedure is over. The surgeon performed it as well as possible, but there is a complication. How to deal with the complication and how it might have been avoided is the purpose of this issue of *Facial Plastic Surgery Clinics of North America*. There is another important consideration, which is the purpose of this article: how will the patient deal with the fact that a complication or untoward result has occurred, and what will be the effect

on the doctor–patient relationship? No patient or surgeon is happy about a complication, and fortunately they are uncommon. However, the patient was not expecting a complication, even though he or she had been informed that it was possible. Informed consent should be detailed and in writing!

It may not be a true complication, but the result is not what the patient (or surgeon) expected. Or perhaps the result is about what the surgeon

Disclosures: The author has no disclosures.
Department of Otolaryngology-Head and Neck Surgery, Stanford Medical Center, 801 Welch Road, Stanford, CA 94305, USA
E-mail address: goode@stanford.edu

Facial Plast Surg Clin N Am 21 (2013) 579–584
http://dx.doi.org/10.1016/j.fsc.2013.07.001
1064-7406/13/$ – see front matter Published by Elsevier Inc.

anticipated but not the patient, a difference in expectations. There is a difference between a true postoperative complication, such as an hematoma or wound infection, and a result that does not meet the patient's expectations.

The latter is more difficult for the surgeon to deal with, because it may be presumed to be caused by the surgeon who did not perform the operation adequately. An infection is not perceived as being caused by the surgeon, whereas a nose that still has some deviation following rhinoplasty or a wide facial scar following a facelift may be perceived as the surgeon's fault.

In addition, the patient's anguish will also depend in part on how easy it will be to fix the problem. A minor office procedure under local anesthesia is a much more acceptable solution than a second procedure under general anesthetic, independent of cost.

The end result is the same, an unhappy patient who wants the surgeon to fix the problem, sooner rather than later. Also in the mix are the questions: "Why did this happen to me?" and "If I had known this would have been the result, I would have never have had the surgery!" And to further compound this issue, what about the case where the surgeon feels the result is good, and the patient does not? Too often, this is the time that the surgeon first realizes he/she has chosen the wrong patient in regard to dealing with an unexpected result.

There are patients who will definitely benefit from facial plastic procedures. They want them done and will pay the surgeon to do so.

But the surgeon should not. Certain patients are easy to pick out as bad psychologic candidates for cosmetic procedures, and I will briefly discuss them. More important are those who are not easy to pick out and reject. This article spends more time on this latter group. The axiom that "the surgeon makes his/her living from the patients on whom he operates while he makes his reputation from those he refuses to operate"[1] is very true, but is hard to do.

Most surgeons have strong egos and are optimistic; they expect to get a good result, and that should produce a happy patient, even in patients who show some signs that they should be rejected as candidates. There is no foolproof method, but experience will provide wisdom on the subject; wisdom is often painfully acquired. Recognizing these patients prior to surgery is an art that must be learned the same as how to do a facelift. But this is only the first part; one must act upon intuition and not do the case. This is harder, particularly in the early years of practice when the economics are extremely important, and a surgeon's rules about on whom not to operate are less defined. Once a medical malpractice suit is filed, the state medical board is asked to suspend the surgeon's license by a patient, or a Web page describes to all what a terrible surgeon one is. The surgeon then will look back and wonder "Should I have seen this coming?"

In addition to over 4 decades of practice, I have benefited from many years as an expert reviewer for the California Medical Board, as well as reviewing some 50 cases of alleged facial plastic surgery medical malpractice for attorneys. So, not only do I have my own experiences in poor patient selection, I have been exposed to those of other surgeons.

Before starting on the categories of patients on whom not to perform surgery, there are some techniques that can help one learn more about patients:

Computer imaging

Computer imaging not only helps make sure the surgeon knows what the patient wants from the surgery but also shows the patient what can realistically be accomplished. It provides another benefit, additional meeting time that allows one to better know the patient prior to any surgery. There are 2 caveats. First, the surgeon must make sure he or she can accomplish the modifications of facial appearance that one provided on the computer-generated images. One should not make it so perfect that the patients' expectations are too high. Second, surgeons are experts in sculpting in flesh but may not be so good when drawing a computer image. If the surgeon does not possess this skill, he or she should learn how to do it or do it outside the presence of the patient and provide it later.

Patients do not like to see their surgeon make a mistake and erase it; I think they worry that a similar error may occur during surgery, and they know that if that happens, it cannot be erased it as it was on the computer images.

Discuss policies regarding fees for revision surgery up front

One's policy on this important matter must be clearly stated to the patient prior to any surgical procedure, preferably in writing. It can be anything the surgeon thinks is fair. Make sure that there is agreement on what is a postoperative result that needs fixing. I tell them we both have to agree that there is a problem following surgery that needs to be fixed and that I am able to fix it. This addresses the point that I must agree there is something that needs to be done, not just the patient. I do not charge a surgical fee for revisions but tell the patient they will have to pay for the use of an operating room and anesthesia, if required. This helps eliminate any "I am not paying for your mistakes" conversations.

PATIENTS WHO ARE EASY TO REJECT

Other Surgeons' Complications

Many surgeons who have been in practice several years spend a sizable percentage of their practice revising cases performed by others where the patient is not happy with the result. These are often difficult cases, and the final result is regularly not perfect. Why would a young surgeon want to do them early in his or her practice when his or her experience is limited? Send them back to the original surgeon. Sometimes the patient will appeal to the surgeon's ego: "I have heard you are the best; I never should have gone to Dr X." Beware...why are they not returning to Dr X? The surgeon should give Dr X a call and tell him/her that the patient is being sent back for further treatment. From Dr X one may find out that "Ms. Y is a crazy lady, and I told her I would not take care of her any longer!" Does the young surgeon really want to do this patient? I recommend at least 10 years in practice before taking on one of these. One's own cases are a different matter.

Litigious Patients

Not a good group. Why would a young surgeon want to do them? There may be reasons, but as stated earlier, I suggest several years in practice before violating this rule. The surgeon may not be aware they have sued a previous surgeon and made his or her life miserable, even if the case went nowhere.

A careful interview by the surgeon or, sometimes better, by an experienced member of the staff may help provide the information. Calling the previous doctor, if known, is usually a good idea, but permission is needed in order to do so.

Patients, for Whatever Reason, the Surgeon (or the Surgeon's Staff) Do Not Like

One needs to determine "why"? Personality? Attitude? Lifestyle? What is It? The surgeon may be wrong, but according to Malcolm Gladwell, who wrote a book titled *Blink*, one's first impression usually turns out to be best.[2] How will the doctor–patient relationship be if there is a postsurgical complication when it starts out with the doctor disliking the patient (and possibly vice versa)? If possible, one should hire an experienced person who has had plastic surgery and is a good evaluator of people. This person may have people skills that the surgeon does not possess and have more time to obtain information that the surgeon did not. This person can discuss costs as well and provide assessment in addition to the surgeon's. If this person does not like the patient, the surgeon should probably not operate.

Patients with a Psychiatric Disorder

Many patients who have had a serious psychiatric illness will not go into detail about it. Suicide attempts, locked ward residence, and other issues may not show up on the medical history sheet. A concern is that the stress of the operation may produce an inappropriate response. Again, a careful history should discover a history of a psychiatric problem but not always. If the patient is seeing a psychiatrist or psychologist, ask the patient for permission to contact that doctor. Refusal should be a red flag to go no further with a surgical option.

Listing the medications a patient is on will help in this regard, and the facial plastic surgeon should be aware of the common (and uncommon) medications used to treat psychiatric illness. Many patients are on antidepressants and this should not, a priori, eliminate them as a candidate. However, the reason for the medications and who is prescribing them should be determined. Patients on haloperidol, lithium, or other medications used to treat major disorders should not be scheduled without psychiatric consultation, in my opinion. It is said that if plastic surgeons eliminate neurotic patients as surgical candidates, they would not have any surgery to do. I have operated on my share, generally with no problems following the surgery. However, certain neurotic traits may be exacerbated by the stress of a postsurgical complication and result in pain to the surgeon as well as the patient.

The patient described by the acronym SIMON for single, immature, male, overexpectant, and narcissistic is another one that deserves increased scrutiny prior to scheduling surgery.[1]

Body Dysmorphic Disorder

This is a psychiatric diagnosis that refers to patients who are so obsessed with a deformity, which may be very minor, that it affects their daily functioning.

These patients may be male or female and of any age, although uncommon in children. They are often depressed with suicidal ideations. Do not operate on these patients.

The Patient with Multiple Medical Comorbidities

This includes patients with significant heart disease, diabetes, poorly controlled hypertension, autoimmune diseases, kidney failure, and patients on long term anticoagulants or with a history of a bleeding disorder. The risk for a postoperative complication is higher in these patients. Minor facial plastic surgery procedures may be well tolerated. Major procedures, however, require a careful preoperative assessment, and I prefer not to do these cases. If the surgeon feels such a patient is a candidate, make sure he or she is medically cleared by the physicians taking care of him or her prior to any procedure and that appropriate monitoring is available during the surgery and in the postoperative period.

PATIENTS DIFFICULT TO EVALUATE

What about those patients who are harder to evaluate as poor candidates for surgery, independent of the defect? Each surgeon will have his or her own bias in regard to the categories listed here. My advice is to be aware of these potential postoperative problem cases that I and other surgeons have identified,[3,4] and over time each surgeon will have his or her own list of whom not to do, which may include additional categories.

The Depressed Patient

One may not be able to tell how depressed a patient is during 1 visit. The usual first clue is found on the standard medical history form where the "depression" box has been checked. In addition, the list of current medications (or allergies) may include more than one antidepressant. Depression is such a common symptom in so many individuals that I feel this category should be considered different from other psychiatric diagnoses. Certainly an adequate history in this area must be taken, ideally by the surgeon or an experienced member of the staff (that older, sage person with great people evaluation skills described earlier).

Be careful of bipolar patients, who may develop a manic or hypomanic phase triggered by a stressful event such as a surgical complication. They may be unreasonable when in this phase and not good patients.

I recommend continued reading regarding assessing patients for personality disorders or psychiatric illness; believe me, it will be worth the time spent. Sending every suspect patient to a psychiatrist for an evaluation prior to surgery is not the answer for most cases; it often makes the patient angry. Furthermore, psychiatrists and psychologists are not infallible; they have malpractice insurance like all physicians and may be wrong when they say a particular patient's psychiatric diagnoses are not a contraindication to facial plastic surgery. Obviously, if they say no surgery, one must follow their advice.

Minor Deformity Patient

First, if one cannot see a real deformity or the patient is fixated on something the surgeon feels is trivial (eg, body dysmorphic disorder), he or she becomes an easy patient not to do. However, minor deformities are usually easier to correct than major ones, and these are some of my best patients. One must ask "Why do you want this corrected?" (which should be part of all preoperative histories). An answer such as "I just lost my job and need to look better" may be true, but if the patient does not find a job after the surgery, will he or she be hypercritical of the surgeon's result? Are the patient's expectations realistic of what the surgeon can do?

Doctor Shoppers

It makes sense to get more than 1 opinion about a planned facial plastic surgery procedure, but there are those who will see 4 or 5 (or more) doctors. I am not sure if there is a magic number, but 3 consultations seems like plenty to me. More than that makes me wonder why the patient needs so many. It may be difficult to find this out, but I do ask each patient if they have seen other doctors.

Those Patients Who Have had Several Plastic Surgery Procedures by Others

Many patients fall into this category, but why now are they coming to a new doctor? There may be a good reason (moved to a new location and heard of the new surgeon) but some may not be so good (sued the last doctor). I recommend calling the other doctor(s) if one can get a name. They may be able to provide helpful information.

The Very Important Person

Watch out. This patient may expect more than the surgeon or staff can provide and become disappointed when the surgeon is unable to provide all the services required. Also, a complication in a high-profile patient may receive much more exposure than the surgeon wants.

The Super Fastidious Patient

Not a hair out of place, make-up perfect, and dress impeccable. May not be a problem patient but will have perfection in mind after surgery and not settle for near perfection, even if the surgeon is happy with the result.

Family Members and Close Friends

Most surgeons have been requested at one time or another to perform facial plastic surgery on family members or close friends. Many surgeons have done this, including me. Still, I do not think this is a good idea. The surgeon's family may not sue over a complication, but feelings of guilt may follow when the surgeon sees the family member who had surgery. Close friends are a treasure; to lose a friendship over a complication is not worth the risk.

Heavy Smokers (Over a Pack a Day)

These patients will have more complications after a facelift. Some surgeons will not do them unless they stop smoking for some finite time period because of poor healing. For other facial plastic surgery procedures, the increased risk of complications is less clear. If possible, one should get patients to stop smoking prior to surgery (difficult to do). Whether this is an absolute contraindication, each surgeon must decide. I think each case should be an individual decision. I have operated on many smokers without incident.

Chronic Pain Patients on Daily Pain Medications

This is another "go slow to schedule" group. If one decides to do them, make sure that the pain medicine prescriber remains in the loop, because postoperative pain control may become a real problem, particularly with a complication. One should determine whether the fee is worth the potential pain problems that may occur with a complication.

Others

The preceding list is not all-inclusive. Several other resources[1,3,4] provide additional information on patient selection.

A COMPLICATION AND AN UNHAPPY PATIENT...NOW WHAT?

Surgical correction has been discussed in other articles in this *Clinics'* publication. I will briefly review some points to help make the patient happy again.

Lots of Hand Holding

Make sure the patient knows the surgeon is concerned and wants to make things right. Having the patient go elsewhere unless the surgeon refers him or her to someone else is not desired. Continue to give the patient follow-up office visits, more than usually needed. I do not charge for these, but I also do not charge for routine postoperative visits even if no complication is present.

Do Everything Possible to Postpone Revision Surgery as Long as—Possible, 1 Year if Possible

I think every surgeon has heard this rule but finds it difficult to follow. The patient pushes the surgeon to fix the problem "now!" "I can't go to work looking like this," and other comments are common. In addition, the surgeon does not want the patient to be a negative advertisement for one's surgical skills. Obviously, some complications can and should be addressed early, such as an opening of a suture line or a subcutaneous fluid collection.

Hopefully, the complication is one that will correct itself or improve over time. That is one important reason to wait. Swelling and scar formation take time to resolve or mature, and early revision surgery may not be able to produce predictable results for this reason. In women, and some men, makeup may be helpful as temporary camouflage, as is a temporary change in hair style.

For Small Depressions or Divots Following Nasal or Facial Surgery, I Inject a Filler as a Temporary Fix

I do not charge for this, but each surgeon's policy on this issue should have been provided prior to surgery. A more permanent fix may be performed later, if still needed.

Occasionally a Referral to a Trusted Colleague Can Help Buy Time

I try to avoid this and only use it rarely. If a surgeon cannot convince a patient to wait, why would the patient be convinced by another surgeon he or she does not know? Besides, the patient will have another bill to pay.

SUMMARY

Finally, the answer on whom not to operate and why becomes clearer and easier to answer the longer one has practiced facial plastic surgery. It is an evolving process, and it takes some 15 to 20 years to really believe in one's intuition (and perhaps that of the staff) that one should say "no" or "not now" to someone who wants one to operate and will pay well. When younger, belief in one's ability dominates, as well as the need to be busy. Later, often after some bad experience, turning down certain patients for surgery becomes easier.

REFERENCES

1. Tardy ME. Rhinoplasty. The art and the science. Philadelphia: W.B. Saunders Company; 1997.
2. Gladwell M. Blink. Boston: Back Bay Books, Little Brown; 2005.
3. The difficult patient. Facial Plast Surg Clin North Am 2008;16:157–276.
4. Goode RL. The unhappy patient following facial plastic surgery: what to do? Facial Plast Surg Clin North Am 2008;16:183–6.

Lasers, Fillers, and Neurotoxins
Avoiding Complications in the Cosmetic Facial Practice

Basil Hassouneh, MD[a], James P. Newman, MD[b],*

KEYWORDS

- Laser resurfacing • Facial fillers • Neurotoxins • Complications in cosmetic surgery

KEY POINTS

- Lasers, injectable fillers, and neurotoxins are extensively used in facial aesthetics.
- Fractional laser resurfacing has introduced a new era in skin rejuvenation, with a lower complication rate and shorter downtime.
- The applications for fillers and neurotoxins have expanded beyond the traditional nasolabial fold correction and forehead lines.
- Permanent and problematic complications can occur, and prompt recognition and appropriate management minimize the sequelae.
- It is the practitioner's understanding of facial anatomy and aesthetic principles that translates the use of these modalities into a safe and pleasing result.

INTRODUCTION

Lasers, injectable fillers, and neurotoxins are widely used in facial restoration and rejuvenation by a variety of practitioners. Although they are less invasive than traditional surgical modalities, they still carry risks for both transient as well as permanent complications. It is paramount for the practitioner to understand these complications, optimize their prevention, and initiate appropriate treatment when they are encountered. This article reviews both early, often transient, complications as well as delayed, often prolonged or permanent, complications with particular focus on prevention and management.

LASER TECHNOLOGIES: SEQUELAE AND COMPLICATIONS

Applications for laser technologies in the practice of facial plastic surgery have expanded. There are several effective modalities for the treatment of aging skin, vascular lesions, telangiectasia, pigmentary irregularities, and acne scarring. Lasers deliver light energy that is absorbed by target tissues (chromophores) to produce photothermal injury. The penetration and energy of the laser, as well as the absorption and thermal relaxation characteristics of the chromophores, dictate the induced thermal injury. In high-energy ablative lasers, the thermolysis involves both the epidermis and the dermis, whereas in low-energy nonablative lasers an intact epidermis cover is spared. The introduction of fractionation has improved the safety of laser resurfacing by using micro pinpoint ablations and allowing the healthy surrounding tissue to accelerate healing.[1,2] Although laser complications can occur following any treatment, there are specific laser and patient factors that contribute to their occurrence (**Table 1**). The American National Standard Institute provides comprehensive details on the safe use of lasers

[a] Health Research Methodology, Department of Clinical Epidemiology & Biostatistics, McMaster University, 1280 Main Street W, Hamilton, ON L8S 4L8, Canada; [b] Stanford University and Premier Plastic Surgery, 1795 El Camino Real, Suite 200, Palo Alto, CA 94306, USA
* Corresponding author.
E-mail address: jnewmanmd@me.com

Facial Plast Surg Clin N Am 21 (2013) 585–598
http://dx.doi.org/10.1016/j.fsc.2013.07.002
1064-7406/13/$ – see front matter © 2013 Elsevier Inc. All rights reserved.

facialplastic.theclinics.com

Table 1
Summary of common laser complications and their management

Complication	Risk Factors	Prevention and Management
Erythema	Sensitive and thin skin Excessive sun damage	Icing, rigorous sun precautions Masking with makeup Treat with topical Biafine (Valeant, Montreal, QC) and 590-nm LED photomodulation Consider a mild topical corticosteroid if condition persists
Blistering and burns	High-energy/penetration lasers Improper pulse stacking or high-density passes Insufficient cooling of the dermis Loss of pain feedback with heavy sedation or general anesthesia	Implement standard device safety and review of laser settings Allow the dermis to cool between passes and after treatment Burn care for severe thermal injuries
Infection and herpetic eruption	Closed facial dressing left >48 h Insufficient facial hygiene/care History of herpetic rash	Adherent to posttreatment facial care with topical disinfectant with hypochlorous acid 0.01% (NeutroPhase, NovaBay, Emeryville, CA) or acetic acid 0.25%–0.0125% (vinegar solution) Prophylactic antibiotic (cephalosporin), and a 1–2 wk anti viral course (valacyclovir) started 24–48 h before treatment
Acne and milia	Closed facial dressings Oil-based creams	Daily facial rinses and noncomedogenic moisturizer Course of oral tetracycline for persistent acne Milia can benefit from topical tretinoin, gentle epidermabrasion, or extraction
Postinflammatory hyperpigmentation	Fitzpatrick skin type III–VI Recent sun exposure/tanning History of hyperpigmented healing	Careful skin type selection with appropriate laser type setting Sun precaution 2–4 wk before treatment and continued for 2–4 mo Prophylactic or therapeutic 2%–4% hydroquinone, 2%–4% kojic acid or Kligman formula (5% hydroquinone, 0.1% tretinoin, and 0.1% dexamethasone). This should be started 2–4 wk before treatment and continued for 2–4 mo
Scarring and hypertrophic healing	Secondary to infections or burns Poor healing capacity History of keloid formation The periorbital region, the neck, and off-face areas	Scar-prone areas require lower fluence and density Apply silicon gel dressing to healing scars and hypertrophic bands Intralesion corticosteroid or 5-fluorouracil

Abbreviation: LED, light-emitting diode.

in health care, and these recommendations should be consulted when setting up a laser procedure room. Standard laser precautions include:

- Adequate signs
- Protective eyewear
- Routine device check with pretesting

There is a risk for ignition whenever high-energy lasers are in use. Accordingly:

- Patients should not have flammable hair sprays or cosmetic products.
- Oxygen supplementation should not flow close to the laser field.
- All flammable tubing should be protected with moist towels.
- Saline should be readily available.

Bruising, Erythema, and Edema

Acute inflammatory skin reaction is an expected sequela following laser treatment. This reaction is generally short-lived and resolves within 2 to 4 days following nonablative treatments and 2 to 4 weeks following ablative treatments. Prolonged erythema beyond these periods is seen in about 1% and 10% of patients, respectively.[3–5] Sensitive plethoric skin, rosacea, and light skin color are more prone to redness. Although women can mask erythema easily with makeup, this is not an attractive option for men. Topical Biafine (Valeant, Montreal, QC) and light-emitting diode photomodulation seem to improve persistent symptoms.[6,7] Hypersensitivity to topical or systemic treatments, albeit difficult to diagnose, should be suspected whenever pruritus or other allergic symptoms are present. Focal edema and exudates can result,

leading to crust formation with small skin breaks, which delays reepithelialization. This problem can be minimized with early icing and liberal moisturizing. Although bruising is rare following routine laser treatment, pulse dye laser is the exception, and patients should be forewarned to better plan the timing of their treatment.[8]

Blistering and Burns

Small blistering occurs particularly with the use of yttrium aluminum garnet (YAG) and Q-switched lasers. These blisters are typically 1 to 2 mm in diameter and can cover the treated area. However, this invariably resolves with no sequelae in 2 to 4 days. Large blisters are more concerning and can indicate significant thermal injury. Insufficient cooling or failure of the cooling system can result in burns of various severities (**Fig. 1**), typically as parallel patches taking the shape of the headpiece. Severe pain is an early indication that heating is excessive, but this important feedback is lost if the procedure is performed under deep sedation or a general anesthetic. Prompt icing and good skin care with daily antiseptic washes can improve the healing of blisters and superficial burns. More extensive injuries are managed in a similar fashion to general burn care.

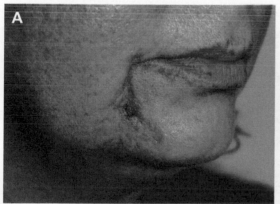
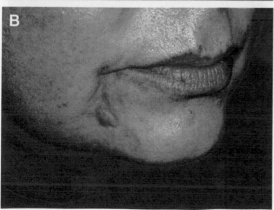
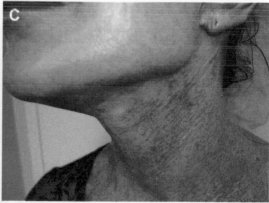

Fig. 1. Patients referred with laser complications. (*A, B*) The healing of hypertrophic scar after pulse stacking with YAG laser for hair removal. (*C*) Permanent hypopigmentation of the face following full ablative skin resurfacing with sharp demarcation line. The effectively treated cheek skin is also smoother and tighter, contrasting with the irregular and relaxed untreated neck.

Infection and Herpetic Eruption

The most common infection after laser skin resurfacing is the reactivation of herpes simplex virus (HSV), with reported rates ranging from 0.5% to 5%.[3] The presence of active lesions is a contraindication to laser treatment. A patient's history of prior HSV eruptions seems unreliable for risk identification. Primary bacterial infections can also occur during the reepithelialization phase. *Staphylococcus aureus* followed by *Pseudomonas aeruginosa* are the most common culprits. *Candida* fungal infections are rare, but have been reported. Many practitioners initiate prophylactic antiviral treatment regardless of the HSV history status. A 1-week to 2-week course of valacyclovir, started 24 to 48 hours before treatment, can decrease the risk for herpetic eruption to less than 0.5%.[9] Some practitioners also initiate prophylactic oral antibiotics (cephalosporin) for 1 week. Spreading cellulitis, purulent discharge, or constitutional symptoms should prompt the physician to obtain cultures for guided antimicrobial therapy. Good facial hygiene is always a critical component of postresurfacing treatment. Open dressing is preferred, because it has the advantage of facilitating early facial care. If a closed dressing is used with deeper resurfacing, it should not be left for more than 48 hours because this increases bacterial growth.[10] The patient should use antiseptic rinses with hypochlorous acid 0.01% (NeutroPhase, NovaBay, Emeryville, CA) or acetic acid 0.25% to 0.0125% (vinegar solution) several times a day until reepithelialization is complete.

Acne and Milia

Acneiform rash erupts following fractional laser treatment in 5% to 10% of cases. Milia represent entrapped hair follicles or sebaceous glands under the reepithelializing skin and usually appear 2 to 3 weeks after treatment. Both conditions seem to be exacerbated with closed facial dressings and oil-based creams. Starting daily facial rinses and noncomedogenic moisturizer can improve these conditions. For patients with a persistent acne flare, a course of oral tetracycline is suitable. Milia can benefit from topical tretinoin, gentle epidermabrasion, or extraction.

Dyschromia

Postinflammatory hyperpigmentation is probably the most common delayed complication (**Fig. 2**) and is rarely permanent.[3–5] It is typically encountered several weeks following ablative CO_2 or Er:YAG laser resurfacing, because the inflammatory healing response leads to epidermal or dermal

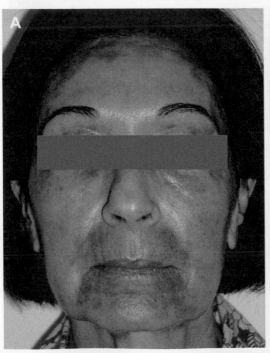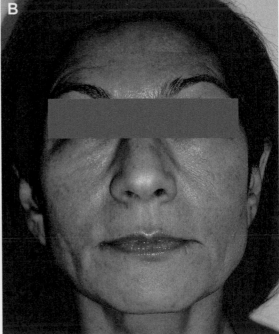

Fig. 2. (*A*) Postinflammatory hyperpigmentation 4 weeks after fractional CO_2 laser resurfacing in a patient with Fitzpatrick skin type IV. (*B*) Twelve weeks after CO_2 laser, now showing resolution after a 3-week course of a 4% hydroquinone topical regimen.

hypermelanosis. Although all skin types can show this inflammatory response, it is almost expected in Fitzpatrick skin types III and greater.[11] The healing behavior of previous wounds or acne sites can also assist in predicting the individual's tendency for hyperpigmented healing. All patients should have strict sun precautions at least 2 to 4 weeks before treatment and continued for at least 2 to 4 months. In high-risk patients, a topical bleaching regimen such as 4% hydroquinone, 2% kojic acid, or Kligman formula (5% hydroquinone, 0.1% tretinoin, and 0.1% dexamethasone) can markedly quiesce melanocytes and is useful for both prevention as well as treatment. Once the desired effect is achieved, a gradual tapering off can minimize rebound. Although hyperpigmentation is temporary, it can persist for several months despite topical treatment. Such patients often show remarkable improvement with superficial chemical peels.

Hypopigmentation is a rare delayed complication that can become evident even several months following treatment and may become permanent.[12] Darker skin tone, previous history of resurfacing, or a prior deep peel are well-recognized risk factors. Demarcation lines, indicating hypopigmentation of the treated skin, were frequently seen with full ablative resurfacing (see **Fig. 1**). However, this is rare in the fractionation era because of the sparing of healthy skin between ablation zones. It is best to address all the aesthetic units of the face with feathering at the borders. This approach provides a smooth transition without abrupt demarcation lines or evident differences in skin texture. Spontaneous repigmentation often takes place over 3 to 4 months. In cases with permanent hypopigmentation, excimer laser, topical photochemotherapy, or alternatively micropigment makeup are all suitable options.[13]

Textural Irregularities

The treatment of isolated facial aesthetic units can accentuate differences in skin texture; this is often seen as smoother, tighter skin in an aggressively treated midface region contrasting with more relaxed and irregular skin over periorbital or lower face regions (see **Fig. 1**). Evident depressions can develop in areas with thin skin and subcutaneous tissue if the deep thermal injury prevents fibroblasts from generating and remodeling collagen. Topical corticosteroids could be a risk factor by suppressing inflammation and fibroblast activity. Infrared or visible-light laser can improve soft irregularities persisting after 6 months by promoting nonablative dermal remodeling. In contrast, autologous fat transfer,

dermal fillers, and subcision are better options for prominent depressions.

Scarring and Hypertrophic Healing

This is a rare complication that is caused by excessive thermal injury or poor healing capacity, or it may be secondary to an infectious complication (see **Fig. 1**). Important patient risk factors include keloid formation, smoking, chronic conditions, or medications that interfere with wound healing. Overly aggressive fluences, high density, insufficient cooling between passes, or improper pulse stacking are all technical factors that can lead to scarring. The periorbital region, the neck, and off-face areas are sensitive and require lower fluence and density.[14,15] If a hypertrophic or keloid scar develops, silicon gel dressing, intralesion corticosteroid, or 5-fluorouracil injection can improve the cosmetic result.

INJECTABLE FILLERS: SEQUELAE AND COMPLICATIONS

A wide variety of injectable materials serve to restore facial volume and soften static wrinkles or folds. It is important for the practitioner to be familiar with the characteristics of each filler and its appropriate use and precautions (**Table 2**). The aesthetic goal for each patient is an individual preference, and should be discussed carefully before treatment. Although many patients come with well-formed desires, it is the practitioner's understanding of facial aging and aesthetic principles that translates the use of fillers into a rejuvenated and pleasing result. Digital photography can aid in documenting pretreatment status, highlighting asymmetries, and detailing facial analysis and goals. In general, complications can arise either from injection trauma or from the filler material. Hyaluronic acid (HA) is the only filler that can be quickly and safely dissolved with enzymatic injection if there is a complication or an undesired result. Hyaluronidase has been used off-label for the last several years with excellent results.[16] Two products approved by the US Food and Drug Administration (FDA) have recently entered the market: Vitrase (Bausch & Lomb, Rochester, NY) and Hylenex (Halozyme Therapeutics, San Diego, CA). This advantage of HA fillers remains significant, particularly for practitioners who are still developing their techniques.

Bruising, Erythema, and Edema

Bruising is the most common complication associated with fillers. Although bruising cannot be eliminated, a variety of measures can decrease the

Table 2
Summary of common fillers and their special characteristics

Filler	Special Characteristics	Precautions
Hyaluronic acid (Juvederm, Allergan, Irvine, CA; Restylane, Medicis, Scottsdale, AZ; Belotero, Merz/BioForm, San Mateo, CA)	Natural molecule across species, provides direct volume restoration Available in different concentrations/cross-linking characteristics: • Thin products used in the superficial dermis • Thick products are used for deeper injections	Negligible risk of allergy (from hyaluronan-associated protein, or bacterial contaminants) No risk of inflammatory nodules; granuloma are rare infectious complication. The only product that can be quickly resolved with enzymatic injection incase of undesirable results Lumpiness and Tyndall effect when placed superficially in areas with thin skin (tear troughs) Belotero advertised to minimize these complications Hyaluronic acid can be enzymatically dissolved with hyalorunidase (Vitrase and Hylenex) Swelling occurs with thick products (not fully hydrated) particularly in high vascular areas such as lips. Icing helps; if socially problematic consider a short course of oral steroid
Poly-L-lactic acid (Sculptra, Valeant, Montreal, QC)	Biocompatible synthetic polymer poly-L-lactic acid in carboxymethylcellulose gel Biostimulatory product with the inflammatory response promoting neocollagenesis	Requires time and several treatments to generate an effect The results can be longer lasting Inflammatory nodules are common (usually palpable but not visible) Avoid superficial injections and overcontracting muscles (orbicularis oculi and orbicularis oris), use higher dilution (8–10 mL total volume per vial), and allow 4 wk between treatments. Nodules usually resolve within a few months; if problematic, try intralesion corticosteroid
Ca hydroxylapatite (Radiesse, Merz/BioForm, San Mateo, CA)	Ca hydroxylapatite (natural component of bone) microspheres suspended in an aqueous carboxymethylcellulose gel carrier Provides immediate filling effect with slow replacement of the carrier gel by neocollagenesis	White filler with thick pasty consistency, not suitable for superficial placement or in areas with thin skin (periorbital region or lips) Occasionally cause nodules that resolve spontaneously
Methylmethacrylate (ArteFill, Suneva San Diego, CA)	Permanent filler composed of nonabsorbable polymethylmethacrylate microspheres suspended in bovine collagen carrier	Recognized risk of allergy to bovine collagen component, and prior skin testing is mandatory Permanent filler and misplacement requires aspiration or surgical excision

(continued on next page)

Table 2
(continued)

Filler	Special Characteristics	Precautions
Liquid silicone	Polydimethylsiloxane is a viscous polymer	Not FDA approved for cosmetic indications (off-label use) Low-grade products have impurities and are not suitable for medical use Permanent filler and misplacement requires aspiration or surgical excision Can cause delayed granuloma reaction (particularly with low-grade silicone products) that is difficult to treat and requires surgical excision

risk. Good understanding of facial vascular anatomy and meticulous avoidance of cutaneous veins are paramount. Applying ice packs before and after injection, using a fine needle (27–28 G) or blunt cannula, and gentle nondistorting pressure can all help avoid unnecessary bruising. Patients are advised to hold medication affecting platelet function 1 week before the injection (nonsteroidal anti inflammatory drugs, aspirin, ginkgo biloba, St John's wort, ginseng, and vitamin E). The patient can also start oral arnica and/or bromelain on the day of the injection; topical arnica may also speed the resolution of bruises. Erythema at the injection site typically represents a short-lived local reaction, although with silicon or collagen fillers this can be a sign of allergic reaction.[17] Edema is expected with the use of non–fully hydrated HA, particularly into highly vascular sites such as the lips. If the patient has unavoidable social demands, a 2-day course of prednisone 50 mg by mouth once a day can control the edema.

Infection and Granuloma

Infection is a rare complication of fillers.[17] Erythema and painful swelling persisting for several days should raise suspicion beyond the usual inflammatory reaction. *S aureus* is the most likely pathogen in the early postinjection period, although HSV reactivation has also been reported. Granulomatous reactions should alert the practitioner to atypical mycobacterial infection or foreign body reaction to the filler material (**Fig. 3**).[18,19] Non–FDA-approved fillers are available in the gray market and abroad; these products have high risk for infections because of bacterial contaminants. The practitioner should have a high degree of suspicion whenever the use of these products is in question. Antiseptic skin preparation and aseptic injection technique are important with all fillers. Overall, infections are treated with

a high-dose cephalosporin or clarithromycin. Temporary fillers usually resolve quickly with the use of hyaluronidase. Patients with a formed abscess or persistent granuloma should undergo drainage, steroid injection, and/or surgical excision.

Violation of Facial Aesthetics

Iatrogenic distortion of aesthetic subunits and contours creates unnatural, inflated, or overdone appearance. Common problems referred to the senior author's practice (J.P. Newman) include so-called moon face from unnatural filling of high cheeks and midface, snout pout from excessive filling of nasolabial folds and white lips, duck lip from disproportional enhancement of the upper lip relative to the lower lip, and sausage lip from loss of the natural cupid's bow and lip contour (**Fig. 4**). Thorough understanding of facial analysis and relations is important to maintain and enhance the aesthetic balance of the face. Good injection technique allows precise delivery of the filler. Graded placement is always a safe approach because it is always easier to add or mold a filler than to remove it. If local infiltration or nerve block is required, small volumes minimize distortion. The patient can continue with gentle massaging after the placement of deep HA fillers or poly-L-lactic acid, but aggressive manipulation can displace the filler.

Lumpiness and Tyndall Effect

The safe placement of a filler requires good appreciation of its physical characteristics, including its drag (G-prime), viscosity, color, and how it scatters light. Lumpiness is felt if thick HA, Ca hydroxylapatite, or poly-L-lactic acid are placed in a superficial plane. Such placement can also create a blue-gray discoloration at the site of injection (known as Tyndall or Rayleigh effect). This discoloration is created because of differences in the

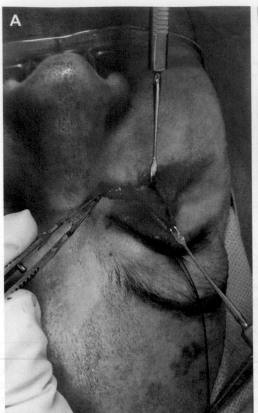
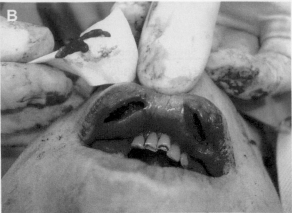
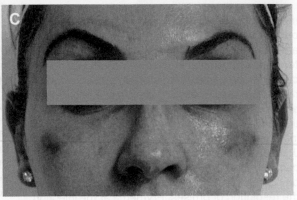

Fig. 3. Patients referred with filler-related complications. (*A*) Reaction fibrosis following Ca hydroxylapatite injection over the infraorbital rim. The patient developed eyelid retraction with tethering to the orbital septum and required surgical excision of the fibrosis. (*B*) Reaction granuloma persisted several years following silicon filler injection to the lips. The patient complained of painful swelling distorting the lip, and required surgical excision. (*C*) Patient referred for chronic edema and hyperpigmentation from overzealous injections of multiple fillers over the midface. Treatment involved topical 4% hydroquinone, sun protection, and observation. ([*A*] *Courtesy of* Dr E.E. Moscato, San Mateo, CA.)

scattering of light depending on its wavelength and the size of the particles encountered.[20] Blue light is scattered 10 times more than red light by large particles, giving rise to an unsightly blue-gray tinge of superficial filler. Areas with thin skin or minimal subcutaneous tissue are at high risk for leaving the filler too superficial, creating lumpiness, Tyndall effect, or both (see **Fig. 4**). These areas include tear troughs, cow's feet, lips, and pucker lines. Belotero (Merz/BioForm, San Mateo, CA) has recently been introduced as an HA filler suitable for superficial placement in these problem areas without significant lumpiness or Tyndall effect.

Biostimulatory fillers such as poly-L-lactic acid and Ca hydroxylapatite can form palpable inflammatory nodules, particularly when placed close to areas of constricting muscle (orbicularis oculi and orbicularis oris).[21–23] The initially high incidence of palpable, but not visible, nodule formation has decreased with increased dilution of

poly-L-lactic acid (1 Sculptra vial rehydrated with 6 mL of sterile preservative free water, then 2 mL of lidocaine 1% are added at the time of injection), and good spacing between treatments (4 weeks). These biostimulatory products are not suitable for the lip or the periorbital region (see **Fig. 3**).

Necrosis and Blindness

Use of fillers is widespread, but there are only a few reports of skin necrosis or blindness complications. These exceedingly rare complications are the most serious events in filler practice. Skin necrosis occurs from injecting the filler material into a facial artery, resulting in embolization to end cutaneous artery or direct occlusion of the vessel, which results in acute ischemia of the skin (**Fig. 5**). The glabellar region carries the highest risk for necrosis, presumable because of the tenuous blood supply and the presence of end-artery vessels coursing abruptly superiorly.[24,25]

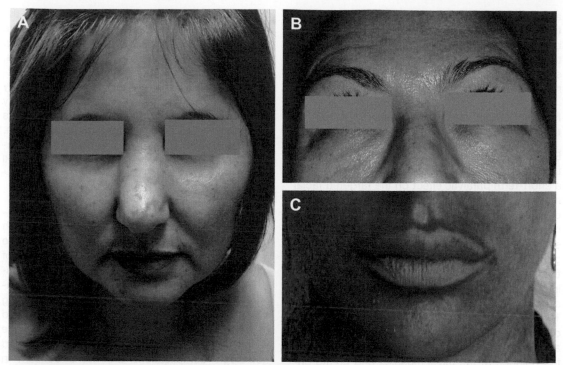

Fig. 4. Patients referred with filler complications. (*A*) Distortion of nasal bridge and brow-tip aesthetic line following HA filler placement to the nose. (*B*) Tyndall effect following placement of thick HA filler to tear troughs. (*C*) Duck-lip appearance from disproportional enhancement of the upper lip relative to the lower lip with HA filler.

Blunt-tip cannula, needle aspiration, retrograde technique, and small-volume filling can all minimize intravascular injections. Special caution should be taken in the anatomic locations of high-risk arteries (supraorbital, supratrochlear, angular, and infraorbital). Pain and pale skin are early signs for end-artery occlusion. In case of HA, prompt treatment with hyaluronidase injection to the site can resolve the acute ischemia. Blindness is another rare but severe complication. It seems to result from retrograde embolization to the ophthalmic artery through the natural

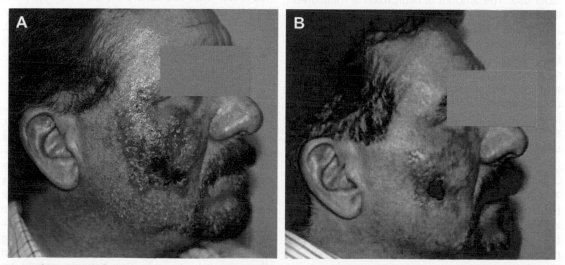

Fig. 5. Skin necrosis following HA filler injection to the cheek. (*A*) Five days after injection, the patient presented with persistent pain and evidence of skin sloughing with superficial infection. (*B*) Five weeks after injection, the patient is showing healing with residual eschar. (*Courtesy of* Dr R. Kassir, Wayne, NJ.)

anastomoses present at the supraorbital, supra-trochlear, or angular arteries. Few cases have been reported to date from various fillers injected to the glabellar or the nasolabial area.[26] Typical symptoms include blindness, pain, and ophthalmoplegia, with poor prognosis for recovery.

NEUROTOXINS: SEQUELAE AND COMPLICATIONS

Botulinum-derived toxins have become a substantial component of facial rejuvenation. They induce a short-term paralytic effect on the targeted facial mimetic muscles to soften unwanted wrinkles, dimples, or bands. Neurotoxins can also produce nonsurgical enhancement of facial aesthetics such as brow lift, square-jaw reduction, and gummy smile correction. The mimetic muscles of the face serve many important functions: expressing language and emotions, handling food and oral secretions, and protecting and lubricating the eye. Therefore, complete loss of movement and tone is often undesirable and leads to a flat, frozen look and interferes with function. It may also alter the balance of the facial muscles and create unnatural dynamic bunching of the orbicularis oculi, abrupt transition of the forehead lines, or secondary muscle recruitment. A balanced conservative treatment plan can avoid many of these consequences and ensure a good aesthetic result (**Table 3**). Botox (Allergan, Irvine, CA) and Dysport (Medicis, Scottsdale, AZ) are both botulinum toxin serotype A and are the only products at present with FDA approval for forehead lines and crow's feet.[27] All other cosmetic uses of neurotoxins, including the perioral region and neck, are off-label use. The amount of neurotoxin is measured in units, and this is determined by the unique L-D50 (the dose of toxin that is lethal in 50% of female Swiss Webster mice per peritoneal injection) of the specific toxin. Although some studies suggested a conversion factor between Botox and Dysport units ranging from 1:3 to 1:5, this is not consistent or reliable in clinical practice.[27] It is best to use the unique units recommended by each manufacturer because the dosing is both site and toxin specific.

Bruising, Erythema, and Edema

The complications encountered from needle trauma are similar to those previously discussed in relation to injectable fillers.[27,28] Bruising is less compared with fillers because of the ultrafine needle caliber, 30 to 32 G, and the superficial muscle target. Injection pain seems to be less when the neurotoxin is reconstituted with preservative-containing saline, compared with preservative-free saline as recommended by the manufacturers.[27,29] Erythema is common at the injection, but this local irritation resolves quickly. Edema sometimes occurs after a few days, typically as puffiness of the eyelids following treatment of the periorbital region. This edema likely reflects lymphatic and venous stasis secondary to paralysis of the orbicularis oculi; cold packs and gentle message can speed the resolution. Hypoanesthesia at the injection site is also common, but this is short-lived and reassurance is all that is needed.

Generalized Effects and Allergic Reactions

Postinjection headache has been associated with neurotoxin injections, and severe migraine-type headaches can be triggered in about 1% of patients. It is unclear whether the neurotoxin is responsible for headaches because a recent meta-analysis showed similar rates in patients receiving saline placebo injections.[30] These patients should receive appropriate analgesics depending on the severity and prior headache history. Cardiac and neurologic complications are not a concern in healthy patients receiving the usual small doses in the cosmetic practice. Neurotoxins are cautioned in pregnancy, lactation, neuromuscular disease (myasthenia gravis, Lambert-Eaton syndrome, and amyotrophic lateral sclerosis), or drugs interacting with the neuromuscular junction (aminoglycosides, calcium channel blockers, cyclosporin A, penicillamine, and quinolones).[27,31] Neutralizing antibodies can develop in 5% of patients, resulting in a decrease in clinical activity.[32] It is usually seen with repeated large total doses; applicable to dystonia rather than cosmetic patients. The antibodies can be against any component of the botulinum toxin protein. Switching to serotype B (Myobloc, Solstice Neurosciences, South San Francisco, CA) resolves this issue because there is no cross reactivity between the serotypes.

Upper Face Iatrogenic Paralysis

Although the unwanted paralysis is temporary, this is one the most unwelcome complications because it can be socially and functionally disruptive for a few months. Iatrogenic paralysis is specific to the site of neurotoxin diffusion and is usually related to improper technique, dosing, or treatment plan. Precise delivery technique with the nondominant hand pressing the target muscle and low-volume, low-pressure injections (diluting 100 Botox units in 1–3 mL) can prevent most of these complications.[33] The patients should be advised to avoid heavy exercise, rubbing of the area, or sleeping face down for 1 day following

Table 3
Summary of common neurotoxin complications and their management

Complications	Risk Factors	Prevention and Management
Bruising	Medication/herbals affecting hemostasis (nonsteroidal anti inflammatory drugs, aspirin, ginkgo biloba, St John's wort, ginseng, and vitamin E)	Discontinue culprit medications/herbals 1 wk before injection Ice packs before and after injection, using a fine needle (27–28 G) or blunt cannula, and gentle nondistorting pressure can all help avoid unnecessary bruising The patient can also start oral arnica and/or bromelain on the day of the injection
	Prominent cutaneous veins	Topical arnica may also speed the resolution of bruises Ultrafine needle gauge, before and after icing, finger pressure
Iatrogenic paralysis:	Generally relates to improper technique, or high-volume, high-pressure injection	Careful planning with patient, correct site and depth, avoid dilute concentration, avoid excessive pressure/messaging
Brow ptosis	Treatment of forehead lines in patients with forehead laxity or brow hooding Preexisting brow ptosis or asymmetry	Avoid lower frontalis; injection 1–1.5 cm above the most inferior forehead line Lower dose in older patients with forehead laxity over the brow or hooding Avoid treatment if there is preexisting brow ptosis masked by the frontalis function
Eyelid ptosis, double vision	Treatment close to supraorbital and orbital rim	Maintain all injections 1 cm outside supraorbital and orbital rims Alpha-adrenergic eye drops (apraclonidine 0.5% or phenylephrine 2.5%) can provide 2 mm of eyelid elevation by stimulating the sympathetically innervated Muller muscle
Lip ptosis	Treatment of orbicularis oculi at the lower eyelid Treatment of nasalis bunny lines	Requires experienced injector. Superficial injections of small dose (1–2 Botox units). Maintain injections medially over the bony nasal pyramid (for the nasalis bunny lines) Maintain injections superior to the inferior orbital rim and boarder of zygoma (for the orbicularis oculi)
Oral incompetency, flattening of cupid's bow	Treatment of perioral rhytides	Requires experienced injector. Injections just outside the vermilion line with no treatment to the central upper lip or corners. Conservative dose to avoid excessive weakness (no more than 2–3 Botox unit to each half lip)
Dysphagia, dysphonia	Treatment of neck platysma bands	Injections superficial to platysma, holding the band with nondominant hand Treatment should not be carried below the superior edge of the thyroid cartilage Few injections per band, spaced 3 cm apart, and maintaining a small total dose (30 Botox units)

treatment to minimize risk of diffusion. Some investigators suggest repeated use of the target muscles 1 hour before injection to improve uptake by the neuromuscular junction. It is important to plan the treatment 1 week before any laser procedures because the edema can increase neurotoxin diffusion.

Brow ptosis is the most common periorbital complication, occurring in about 3% to 5% of patients when treating the forehead lines.[34,35] A high degree of soft tissue laxity over the brow or hooding is an important risk factor. Asking the patient to close their eyes, holding the frontalis with the examiner's hand, then asking the patient to open their eyes can provide good assessment of expected brow position without the frontalis function. This technique is particularly useful to unmask preexisting brow ptosis. As a general principle, injections should be at least 1 to 1.5 cm above the most inferior forehead line. The dose should be adjusted according to the individual patient. Chemical contouring of the brow is an attractive option for many patients and can provide desirable arching or flaring when performed by an experienced practitioner. Evaluation of brow position on each side is important to avoid exacerbating a preexisting asymmetry. The orbicularis oculi is important for blinking and maintaining lid opposition against the globe. Assessment of lower lid tissues with snap test and distraction test can screen patients who are at risk for ectropion and dry eyes. In general, a small dose (1–2 Botox units) per injection site is sufficient for treatments along the brow and in the crow's feet area because the orbicularis oculi muscle is thin. Directing the needle away from the eye is a safe technique not only to protect the globe from unexpected movements but also to avoid inadvertent injections medial to the orbital rims. The injection should always be at least 1 cm away from the bony orbital rims to avoid possible diffusion to the levator palpebrae or the ocular muscles. Although higher complication rates have been reported, the occurrence of lid ptosis or diplopia is usually less than 1% in the hands of experienced practitioner.[34,35] Ocular complications are bothersome because they interfere with the patient's vision. Alpha-adrenergic eye drops (apraclonidine 0.5% or phenylephrine 2.5%) can provide 2 mm of eyelid elevation by stimulating the sympathetically innervated Muller muscle.

Midface and Lower Face Iatrogenic Paralysis

Treatment of the perioral region is associated with a high rate of complications. An experienced practitioner and conservative dosing are both important to minimize undesirable effects. Lip ptosis or smile asymmetry can result from diffusion of neurotoxin to the levators of the lip or the zygomaticus major muscle, which usually occurs when treating the nasalis bunny lines or the orbicularis oculi at the lower eyelid. Injections should be superficial in these sites and maintained medially over the bony nasal pyramid (for the nasalis bunny lines) and superior to the inferior orbital rim and boarder of the zygoma (for the lower eyelid orbicularis oculi). The dose should be conservative (1–2 Botox units) because these muscles are thin.

Neurotoxin can offer effective treatment to perioral rhytides, often called smoker's lines. These vertical rhytides can be softened with small doses (no more than 2 to 3 Botox units to each half lip) delivered just outside the vermilion line. If the central part of the upper lip is treated, the cupid's bow becomes flat.[36] These treatments can also affect lip competency and should be cautioned in singers or those with specific instrument demands. Neck platysma bands respond well to neurotoxin treatment. The treatment should not be carried below the superior edge of the thyroid cartilage. The target is the platysma; holding the muscle band with the nondominant hand can facilitate precise depth of injection. Few injections per band spaced 3 cm apart while maintaining a small total dose (30 Botox units) can avoid potential dysphagia or dysphonia from diffusion of the neurotoxin to the deeper pharyngeal or laryngeal muscles.[36]

SUMMARY

Lasers, injectable fillers, and neurotoxins are widely used in facial aesthetics. Fractional laser resurfacing has introduced a new era in skin rejuvenation, with lower complication rates and shorter downtime. Applications for fillers and neurotoxins have also expanded beyond the traditional nasolabial fold correction and forehead lines. These products continue to show steady growth in the number of patients treated each year. With this expansion in clinical practice, becoming familiar with potential complications and their management is paramount. Although most complications are temporary and minor, permanent and problematic complications can occur. Prevention is always the best approach, but prompt recognition and appropriate management minimize the sequelae. Many products and technologies are now available in the armamentarium of facial plastic surgery. It is the practitioner's understanding of facial anatomy and aesthetic principles that translates the use of these modalities into a safe and pleasing result.

ACKNOWLEDGMENTS

The authors thank Dr Eve E. Moscato for providing photographs of reaction fibrosis with eyelid retraction following filler injection, and Dr Ramtin Kassir for providing photographs of skin necrosis following filler injection.

REFERENCES

1. Saedi N, Petelin A, Zachary C. Fractionation: a new era in laser resurfacing. Clin Plast Surg 2011;38(3): 449–61, vii.

2. Taub AF. Fractionated delivery systems for difficult to treat clinical applications: acne scarring, melasma, atrophic scarring, striae distensae, and deep rhytides. J Drugs Dermatol 2007;6(11):1120–8.

3. Graber EM, Tanzi EL, Alster TS. Side effects and complications of fractional laser photothermolysis: experience with 961 treatments. Dermatol Surg 2008;34(3):301–5 [discussion: 305–7].

4. Rahman Z, MacFalls H, Jiang K, et al. Fractional deep dermal ablation induces tissue tightening. Lasers Surg Med 2009;41(2):78–86.

5. Fisher GH, Geronemus RG. Short-term side effects of fractional photothermolysis. Dermatol Surg 2005; 31(9 Pt 2):1245–9 [discussion: 1249].

6. Sarnoff DS. A comparison of wound healing between a skin protectant ointment and a medical device topical emulsion after laser resurfacing of the perioral area. J Am Acad Dermatol 2011;64(Suppl 3):S36–43.

7. Alster TS, Wanitphakdeedecha R. Improvement of postfractional laser erythema with light-emitting diode photomodulation. Dermatol Surg 2009;35(5): 813–5.

8. Alam M, Dover JS, Arndt KA. Treatment of facial telangiectasia with variable-pulse high-fluence pulsed-dye laser: comparison of efficacy with fluences immediately above and below the purpura threshold. Dermatol Surg 2003;29(7):681–4 [discussion: 685].

9. Beeson WH, Rachel JD. Valacyclovir prophylaxis for herpes simplex virus infection or infection recurrence following laser skin resurfacing. Dermatol Surg 2002;28(4):331–6.

10. Newman JP, Koch RJ, Goode RL. Closed dressings after laser skin resurfacing. Arch Otolaryngol Head Neck Surg 1998;124(7):751–7.

11. Chan HH, Manstein D, Yu CS, et al. The prevalence and risk factors of post-inflammatory hyperpigmentation after fractional resurfacing in Asians. Lasers Surg Med 2007;39(5):381–5.

12. Tierney EP, Hanke CW. Treatment of CO_2 laser induced hypopigmentation with ablative fractionated laser resurfacing: case report and review of the literature. J Drugs Dermatol 2010;9(11):1420–6.

13. Alexiades-Armenakas MR, Bernstein LJ, Friedman PM, et al. The safety and efficacy of the 308-nm excimer laser for pigment correction of hypopigmented scars and striae alba. Arch Dermatol 2004;140(8):955–60.

14. Avram MM, Tope WD, Yu T, et al. Hypertrophic scarring of the neck following ablative fractional carbon dioxide laser resurfacing. Lasers Surg Med 2009; 41(3):185–8.

15. Lee SJ, Kim JH, Lee SE, et al. Hypertrophic scarring after burn scar treatment with a 10,600-nm carbon dioxide fractional laser. Dermatol Surg 2011;37(8): 1168–72.

16. Hirsch RJ, Brody HJ, Carruthers JD. Hyaluronidase in the office: a necessity for every dermasurgeon that injects hyaluronic acid. J Cosmet Laser Ther 2007;9(3):182–5.

17. Zielke H, Wolber L, Wiest L, et al. Risk profiles of different injectable fillers: results from the Injectable Filler Safety Study (IFS Study). Dermatol Surg 2008; 34(3):326–35 [discussion: 335].

18. Toy BR, Frank PJ. Outbreak of *Mycobacterium abscessus* infection after soft tissue augmentation. Dermatol Surg 2003;29(9):971–3.

19. Christensen L. Normal and pathologic tissue reactions to soft tissue gel fillers. Dermatol Surg 2007; 33(Suppl 2):S168–75.

20. Hirsch RJ, Narurkar V, Carruthers J. Management of injected hyaluronic acid induced Tyndall effects. Lasers Surg Med 2006;38(3):202–4.

21. Rendon MI. Long-term aesthetic outcomes with injectable poly-l-lactic acid: observations and practical recommendations based on clinical experience over 5 years. J Cosmet Dermatol 2012;11(2): 93–100.

22. Fitzgerald R, Vleggaar D. Facial volume restoration of the aging face with poly-l-lactic acid. Dermatol Ther 2011;24(1):2–27.

23. Tzikas TL. A 52-month summary of results using calcium hydroxylapatite for facial soft tissue augmentation. Dermatol Surg 2008;34(Suppl 1):S9–15.

24. Glaich AS, Cohen JL, Goldberg LH. Injection necrosis of the glabella: protocol for prevention and treatment after use of dermal fillers. Dermatol Surg 2006; 32(2):276–81.

25. Kassir R, Kolluru A, Kassir M. Extensive necrosis after injection of hyaluronic acid filler: case report and review of the literature. J Cosmet Dermatol 2011; 10(3):224–31.

26. Park SW, Woo SJ, Park KH, et al. Iatrogenic retinal artery occlusion caused by cosmetic facial filler injections. Am J Ophthalmol 2012;154(4):653–62.e1.

27. Berry MG, Stanek JJ. Botulinum neurotoxin A: a review. J Plast Reconstr Aesthet Surg 2012;65(10): 1283–91.

28. Cote TR, Mohan AK, Polder JA, et al. Botulinum toxin type A injections: adverse events reported to the US

Food and Drug Administration in therapeutic and cosmetic cases. J Am Acad Dermatol 2005;53(3): 407–15.

29. Sarifakioglu N, Sarifakioglu E. Evaluating effects of preservative-containing saline solution on pain perception during botulinum toxin type-a injections at different locations: a prospective, single-blinded, randomized controlled trial. Aesthetic Plast Surg 2005;29(2):113–5.

30. Brin MF, Boodhoo TI, Pogoda JM, et al. Safety and tolerability of onabotulinumtoxinA in the treatment of facial lines: a meta-analysis of individual patient data from global clinical registration studies in 1678 participants. J Am Acad Dermatol 2009; 61(6):961–70.e1–11.

31. Huang W, Foster JA, Rogachefsky AS. Pharmacology of botulinum toxin. J Am Acad Dermatol 2000;43(2 Pt 1):249–59.

32. Benecke R. Clinical relevance of botulinum toxin immunogenicity. BioDrugs 2012;26(2):e1–9.

33. Hsu TS, Dover JS, Arndt KA. Effect of volume and concentration on the diffusion of botulinum exotoxin A. Arch Dermatol 2004;140(11):1351–4.

34. Carruthers JA, Lowe NJ, Menter MA, et al. A multicenter, double-blind, randomized, placebo-controlled study of the efficacy and safety of botulinum toxin type A in the treatment of glabellar lines. J Am Acad Dermatol 2002;46(6):840–9.

35. Vartanian AJ, Dayan SH. Complications of botulinum toxin A use in facial rejuvenation. Facial Plast Surg Clin North Am 2005;13(1):1–10.

36. Raspaldo H, Niforos FR, Gassia V, et al. Lower-face and neck antiaging treatment and prevention using onabotulinumtoxin A: the 2010 multidisciplinary French consensus–part 2. J Cosmet Dermatol 2011;10(2):131–49.

Complications in Facial Flap Surgery

Charles R. Woodard, MD

KEYWORDS

- Facial flap • Complications • Mohs reconstruction • Tension • Ischemia • Hematoma • Infection

KEY POINTS

- Local facial flaps are commonly used to reconstruct facial defects.
- Complications of facial flaps include those of tension-related, ischemic, hematologic, and infectious etiology.
- Complication avoidance is achieved through thorough patient evaluation, thoughtful preoperative planning, and meticulous surgical technique.

INTRODUCTION

The American Cancer Society estimates an incidence of approximately 3.5 million cases of nonmelanoma skin cancer in the past year.[1] Of these, the majority occur in the sun-exposed head and neck. From 1992 to 2006 the treatment of nonmelanoma skin cancer increased by 77%.[2] Consequently, the number of facial reconstructions performed also increased.

Local flaps are the criterion standard for reconstruction of most cutaneous defects of the face. Complications from these procedures are readily apparent given the sensitive location of the surgical repair. Depending on the area treated, the complication may result in functional and/or aesthetic sequelae.

Complications from local flap reconstruction result from tension-related, ischemic, hematologic, and infectious causes. Such complications may arise intraoperatively or may not occur until the early or late postoperative phases. Prevention of complications is based on the surgeon's understanding of the fundamental principles of facial reconstruction. Selection of the appropriate technique is critical to a successful outcome. The mutual goal is a balanced functional and aesthetic result that is pleasing to the patient as well as the

surgeon. This result is accomplished through a systematic, comprehensive analysis of defects. The surgeon must consider the following questions when developing the reconstructive plan[3]:

1. Which surrounding landmarks must not be distorted or subject to tension by the reconstruction?
2. Where is the vector of tension created during flap inset as well as throughout the normal healing process?
3. What region of tissue recruitment offers maximal laxity?
4. How are the relaxed skin-tension lines and borders of aesthetic subunits oriented?
5. Is the blood supply of the designed flap adequate?

EVALUATION OF THE PATIENT

Avoidance of complications begins in the preoperative period with a thorough patient history and physical examination. A standardized medical screening questionnaire is often useful in identifying pertinent medical history that may predispose a patient to otherwise unanticipated complications. Hypertension, diabetes, liver failure, immune suppression, renal failure, inherited blood dyscrasias,

There are no relevant financial disclosures.
Division of Otolaryngology-Head & Neck Surgery, Facial Plastic and Reconstructive Surgery, Duke University Medical Center, DUMC 3805, Durham, NC 27710, USA
E-mail address: charles.woodard@duke.edu

inflammatory skin conditions, history of hypertrophic scarring/keloids, and prior radiation exposure can all negatively affect the surgical result.[4,5]

Many surgeons elicit a history on prescription medications including nonsteroidal anti-inflammatories and antiplatelet therapies, given their known effects on coagulation. However, herbal supplements are sometimes overlooked. Popular supplements, including ginkgo biloba, garlic, ginger, ginseng, feverfew, vitamin E, licorice, bilberry, German chamomile, red clover, poplar, meadowsweet, willowbark, tamarind, turmeric, danshen, dong quai, alfalfa, goldenseal, and green tea, should receive special consideration given their effects on the clotting cascade.[6–8]

Use of alcohol and tobacco increases the risk of complications following surgery. Heavy alcohol use affects the hepatic system, which in turn affects both the clotting cascade and drug metabolism.[9] Tobacco use has a well-documented detrimental effect on tissue perfusion.[10,11] Nicotine adversely affects tissue perfusion while carbon monoxide lowers cutaneous oxygenation. Heavy smokers (greater than 1 pack per day) have a 3 times higher incidence of postoperative flap necrosis.[12]

TENSION-RELATED COMPLICATIONS

Achieving a tension-free closure is fundamental to surgical success. Excess tension may serve as the catalyst for development of ischemic,

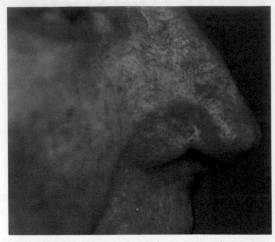

Fig. 1. Alar retraction after advancement flap repair. (*Courtesy of* Sam Most, MD, Stanford University Medical Center, Stanford, CA.)

hematologic, and infectious complications. Placement of incisions parallel to relaxed skin-tension lines and along aesthetic subunit borders allows for maximal extensibility and camouflage of the resultant scar.

In addition, tension must not distort the immobile surrounding landmarks. The nose, eyelids, and lips are particularly susceptible to this distortion (**Figs. 1–3**). With respect to the nose, the superior vector of alar retraction and tip twisting is well recognized. However, there remains an

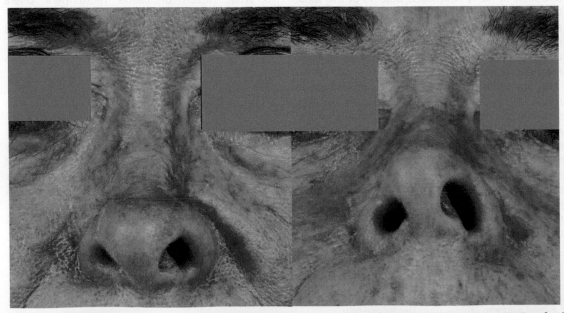

Fig. 2. Twisted tip following local flap and full-thickness skin-graft repair. (*Courtesy of* Sam Most, MD, Stanford University Medical Center, Stanford, CA.)

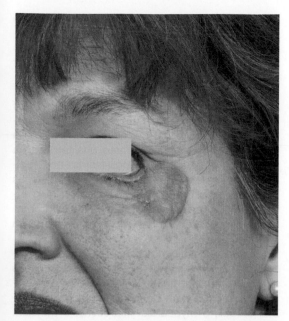

Fig. 3. Ectropion after cheek advancement flap and full-thickness skin-graft repair. (*Courtesy of* Sam Most, MD, Stanford University Medical Center, Stanford, CA.)

additional perpendicular tension vector requiring consideration. As the wound bed contracts, it tends to draw the flap medially or intranasally. This problem is significant for reconstructions overlying the ala or supra-alar crease, as a medial displacement in this region will tend to narrow the nasal valve and may lead to iatrogenic nasal obstruction.[13]

Pincushioning is a complication seen in facial reconstruction (**Fig. 4**) that occurs as a result of contraction of the flap and lymphedema of the wound edge. Reconstructions of the nose are particularly susceptible to this problem for 2 reasons. First, the available surrounding donor tissue is more limited than other facial subunits. Second, the quality and texture of the nasal skin changes significantly from thin skin at the rhinion to thick, sebaceous skin along the tip. This factor must be taken into consideration when designing flaps that transition across these different textural areas of the nose. Ensuring a tension-free closure with appropriate eversion of the wound edges will help reduce pincushioning.

ISCHEMIC COMPLICATIONS

The face enjoys a rich blood supply. Under normal conditions, blood flow is approximately 10 times that needed to provide adequate nutritional support[14]; however, under conditions of stress the flow is less predictable. Blood flow depends on

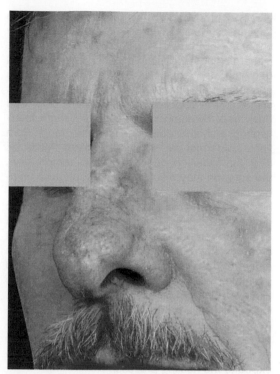

Fig. 4. Pincushioning of a nasal bilobe flap. (*Courtesy of* Sam Most, MD, Stanford University Medical Center, Stanford, CA.)

a coordination of precapillary sphincters and arteriovenous shunts that direct arteriolar perfusion pressure.[15] The flow is driven through major distributing vessels, along septocutaneous and musculocutaneous perforators, and into a dense interconnecting network of dermal and subdermal plexuses. This redundancy in blood supply allows for successful design of random flaps, which account for the majority of local facial flap reconstructions.[16]

Delicate technique and proper flap design are the cornerstones of a successful surgical result. Technical aspects of the procedure include tissue handling, adequate undermining, and suture placement. Toothed forceps and skin hooks can cause damage to the flap margins, leading to ischemic compromise. Adequate undermining is essential to a tension-free closure. As the flap's blood supply is inversely proportional to the distance from the base of the flap, it is important that undue tension is prevented, especially along the distal aspect of the flap.

Consideration of expected postoperative edema is important when placing sutures along the wound edge, as they may strangulate portions of the flap if secured too tightly.

Following inset, a pale flap with slow capillary refill heralds impending ischemia. If recognized intraoperatively, additional undermining to relieve tension or modification of suture technique may improve the blood flow at the wound edge. Ischemic flaps secondary to poor flap design will demonstrate ischemia before inset. Venous congestion may also lead to flap ischemia, and is suspected in flap edema with a dark color and brisk dark bleeding with pinprick. Without intervention, ischemic consequences may range from flap epidermolysis to full-thickness necrosis (**Fig. 5**). If there is concern for flap compromise, the surgeon may elect to use intraoperative angiography to objectively evaluate flap perfusion.[17]

Management of tissue loss from ischemic changes is often conservative. The surgeon should avoid the temptation to initially debride suspect areas of the reconstruction. Depending on the extent of tissue loss, when left to heal by second intention, an acceptable result is sometimes achieved without further intervention (**Fig. 6**). Once the tissue has declared its viability, devitalized tissue that is easily removed may be debrided. Judicious wound care to include an antibiotic emollient and frequent cleaning may expedite the healing process.

HEMATOLOGIC COMPLICATIONS

Most hematologic complications in local flap surgery result from drug-induced coagulopathy and/or inadequate intraoperative hemostasis.[18] In addition, appropriate perioperative control of blood pressure will reduce the risk of hematoma formation. In cases where the anticoagulation plan is unclear or the patient has uncontrolled hypertension, surgical delay is prudent until these problems are solved.

In a meta-analysis of cutaneous surgery, Lewis and Dufresne[19] found a 6-fold increased risk of moderate to severe bleeding complications in patients taking warfarin (Coumadin) (12.3% vs 2.1%). Aspirin produced a nonsignificant increased risk of bleeding with a 4% moderate to severe complication rate. Definitions of "moderate" and "severe" in these studies were variable and qualitative. In a retrospective study by Cook-Norris and colleagues,[20] severe complications were 6 times more likely with clopidogrel (Plavix)-containing anticoagulation, and 8 times more likely with combined clopidogrel and aspirin than with aspirin monotherapy.

Cessation of anticoagulation may lead to thrombotic complications. In a survey of 168 Mohs surgeons, 49 thrombotic complications were reported in 46 patients (3 deaths, 24 strokes, 3 cerebral emboli, 5 myocardial infarctions, 8 transient ischemic attacks, 3 deep vein thrombosis, 2 pulmonary emboli, and 1 retinal artery occlusion).[21] Fifty-four percent were attributed to aspirin discontinuation and 39% to withholding warfarin. It is clear that these complications are significantly more morbid than bleeding complications that result from continuation of these medications. Therefore, the surgeon must have a thorough discussion with the prescribing physician regarding adequate management of perioperative anticoagulation.

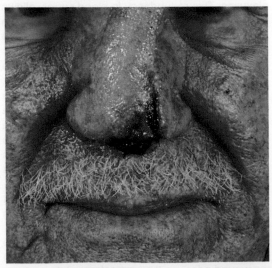

Fig. 5. Epidermolysis of the distal aspect of the forehead flap demarcated by a preexisting forehead scar incorporated in the flap. (*Courtesy of* Sam Most, MD, Stanford University Medical Center, Stanford, CA.)

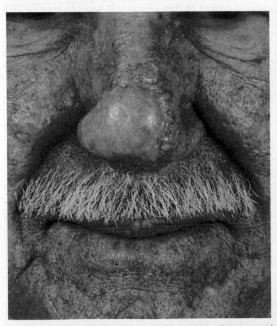

Fig. 6. Surgical result 1 month after aggressive wound care and second-intention healing. (*Courtesy of* Sam Most, MD, Stanford University Medical Center, Stanford, CA.)

Intraoperatively, hemorrhage is averted with meticulous hemostasis. The addition of epinephrine to local anesthetic helps minimize bleeding in the surgical field, but the surgeon must allow adequate time for effect. Bleeding complications are most likely to occur during the initial incision or undermining of the tissue adjacent the wound.[22] A thorough understanding of the underlying anatomy will directly reduce the risk of this complication. Undermining in a uniform plane at the correct depth minimizes blood loss. Vessel identification with judicious use of electrocautery allows for a relatively bloodless field. In cases of hemorrhage, it is essential to accurately identify the source of bleeding to reduce iatrogenic damage to the surrounding tissues.

Postoperative pressure dressings may provide an additional measure of hemostasis, although they are often challenging to place on the face. In addition, too much pressure may lead to an ischemic complication. It is best to ensure hemostasis before flap inset to reduce the risk of complication.

Early recognition of hematoma formation requires a high index of suspicion in the perioperative period. Flaps that are tense and demonstrate a change in color often indicate hematoma formation. An increase in pain is often a harbinger of a developing hematoma. If recognized early, aspiration with a large-bore needle (eg, 18-gauge) and application of pressure may help. The surgeon should have a low threshold for return to the operative suite for wound exploration, hematoma evacuation, and identification of the bleeding source if conservative measures do not control the bleeding.

INFECTIOUS COMPLICATIONS

Postsurgical infection rates for clean-wound facial surgery remain low, at approximately 3%.[23] Clean-contaminated wounds of the oral cavity and intranasal mucosa carry a slightly higher risk of infection. Infection is best managed using preventive strategies including antiseptics and aseptic techniques. In clean wounds, which represent the majority of facial flap procedures, prophylactic antibiotics are not indicated.[24] Antibiotics for clean-contaminated wounds are more controversial.

A combination of induration, erythema, and wound warmth may indicate an infection. The patient may or may not present with a fever. Purulent drainage should be cultured. The most common organisms isolated from these wounds include *Staphylococcus aureus*, coagulase-negative staphylococci, and *Pseudomonas*. As most infections are bacterial in nature, antibiotics should be initiated. Empiric therapy is often with antistaphylococcal antibiotics. Unfortunately, there is an increasing incidence of both community-acquired and hospital-acquired methicillin-resistant *S aureus*, which the surgeon must therefore consider in infections that do not improve with standard treatment.

SUMMARY

Complications are an expected consequence of surgical intervention, and facial flaps are no exception. The goal is to recognize and avoid pitfalls that lead to such complications. A comprehensive preoperative evaluation, well-developed reconstruction plan, and thorough understanding of flap design and execution will minimize complication rates.

REFERENCES

1. American Cancer Society. Detailed guide: skin cancer: basal and squamous cell. Available at: http://www.cancer.org/cancer/skincancer-basalandsquamouscell/detailedguide/index. Accessed November 2, 2012.
2. Rogers HW, Weinstock MA, Harris AR, et al. Incidence estimate of nonmelanoma skin cancer in the United States, 2006. Arch Dermatol 2010;146(3):283–7.
3. Park SS. Cutaneous lesions and facial reconstruction. In: Park SS, editor. Facial plastic surgery: the essential guide. New York: Thieme; 2005. p. 61–115.
4. Salasche SJ, Grabski WJ. Complications of flaps. J Dermatol Surg Oncol 1991;17:132–40.
5. Peterson SR, Joseph AK. Inherited bleeding disorders in dermatologic surgery. Dermatol Surg 2001; 27:885–9.
6. Chang LK, Whitaker DC. The impact of herbal medicines on dermatologic surgery. Dermatol Surg 2001;27:759–63.
7. Dinehart SM, Henry L. Dietary supplements: altered coagulation and effects on bruising. Dermatol Surg 2005;31:819–26.
8. Collins SC, Dufresne RG. Dietary supplements in the setting of Mohs surgery. Dermatol Surg 2002;28: 447–52.
9. Salem RO, Laposata M. Effects of alcohol on hemostasis. Am J Clin Pathol 2005;123(Suppl 1): S96–105.
10. Kinsella JB, Rassekh CH, Wassamuth ZD, et al. Smoking increases skin flap complications. Ann Otol Rhinol Laryngol 1999;108:139–42.
11. Vural E, Key JM. Complications, salvage, and enhancement of local flaps in facial reconstruction. Otolaryngol Clin North Am 2001;4:739–51.
12. Goldminz D, Bennett RG. Cigarette smoking and flap and full-thickness graft necrosis. Arch Dermatol 1991;127:1012–5.

13. Woodard CR, Park SS. Reconstruction of nasal defects 1.5 cm or smaller. Arch Facial Plast Surg 2011;13(2):97–102.

14. Goding GS, Hom DB. Skin flap physiology. In: Baker SR, editor. Local flaps in facial reconstruction. Philadelphia: Mosby; 1995. p. 15–30.

15. Sherman J. Normal arteriovenous anastomoses. Medicine 1963;42:247–67.

16. Honrado CP, Murakami CS. Wound healing and physiology of skin flaps. Facial Plast Surg Clin North Am 2005;13:203–14.

17. Woodard CR, Most SP. Intraoperative angiography using laser-assisted indocyanine green imaging to map perfusion of forehead flaps. Arch Facial Plast Surg 2012;14(4):263–9.

18. Zoumalan RA, Murakami CS. Facial flap complications. Facial Plast Surg 2012;28(3):347–53.

19. Lewis KG, Dufresne RG Jr. A meta-analysis of complications attributed to anticoagulation among patients following cutaneous surgery. Dermatol Surg 2008;34(2):160–4.

20. Cook-Norris RH, Michaels JD, Weaver AL, et al. Complications of cutaneous surgery in patients taking clopidogrel-containing anticoagulation. J Am Acad Dermatol 2011;65(3):584–91.

21. Kovich O, Otley CC. Thrombotic complications related to discontinuation of warfarin and aspirin therapy perioperatively for cutaneous operation. J Am Acad Dermatol 2003;48(2):233–7.

22. Bunick CG, Aasi SZ. Hemorrhagic complications in dermatologic surgery. Dermatol Ther 2007;24(6):537–50.

23. Sylaidis P, Wood S, Murray DS. Postoperative infection following clean facial surgery. Ann Plast Surg 1997;39:342–6.

24. Wood LD, Warner NM, Billingsley EM. Infectious complications of dermatologic procedures. Dermatol Ther 2011;24:558–70.

Complications in Facial Trauma

Lisa M. Morris, MD, Robert M. Kellman, MD*

KEYWORDS

- Facial trauma • Complications • Orbit • Zygomaticomaxillary complex • Nasoorbitoethmoid
- Mandible

KEY POINTS

- Intracranial and ocular injuries are common with severe facial fractures, and must be quickly identified and appropriately treated.
- Meticulous fracture reduction and implant placement are paramount in preventing postoperative complications.
- Complications of rigid fixation are typically due to fixation of inadequately reduced fractures.
- Close postoperative assessment allows for early recognition of complications, and provides the opportunity to intervene when necessary to achieve better long-term outcomes.

INTRODUCTION

Complications are common in the facial trauma setting, and there are several causes. All facial trauma surgeons should be knowledgable about potential associated intracranial and ocular injuries and how to prevent further morbidity. A multidisciplinary approach is often required, and early consultation with appropriate specialists is recommended. An understanding of common posttraumatic complications will guide surgical management. The most common complications of facial trauma are summarized in **Tables 1** and **2**.

SURGICAL COMPLICATIONS OF SOFT TISSUE AND VISCERA

Important overall tenets of facial trauma are to minimize scarring and prevent further injury to adjacent structures. The bony skeleton of the face protects multiple organs that are important to the functions of daily life. It is imperative that these organs are thoroughly evaluated at the initial presentation and the findings accurately

documented. Scarring may be unavoidable, depending on the damage to soft tissue from the primary injury and/or location of the fractures and the access required for their repair. Lacerations should be copiously irrigated, minimally debrided, and closed primarily in a layered fashion.[1] Local skin flaps may be used to cover defects, if necessary. Hypertrophic or cosmetically unfavorable scars can be treated with dermabrasion, serial excision, or scar revision.

Brain injuries occur in up to 89% of patients with complex facial trauma.[2] All patients should be evaluated for potential involvement of the brain or cervical spine (**Table 3**), and an urgent neurosurgical consultation should be obtained for any positive findings. Traumatic brain injuries can be classified as closed, penetrating, and explosive blast injuries, with the severity based on the Glasgow Coma Scale.[3] Cerebrospinal fluid (CSF) leaks carry a 10% to 30% risk of developing meningitis, and can present acutely at the time of initial injury or in a delayed fashion.[4,5] Symptoms include persistent clear rhinorrhea or otorrhea, description of a salty taste in the mouth by the patient,

Department of Otolaryngology & Communication Sciences, Upstate Medical University, State University of New York, 750 East Adams Street, Syracuse, NY 13210, USA
* Corresponding author.
E-mail address: kellmanr@upstate.edu

Facial Plast Surg Clin N Am 21 (2013) 605–617
http://dx.doi.org/10.1016/j.fsc.2013.07.005
1064-7406/13/$ – see front matter © 2013 Elsevier Inc. All rights reserved.

facialplastic.theclinics.com

Table 1
Complications of facial trauma: soft tissue and viscera

	Early	Late/Postoperative
Soft tissue	Infection/abscess Loss of soft tissue Unfavorable scarring	Scar contracture Facial deformity Infection/abscess
Brain	Dural laceration Cerebrospinal fluid (CSF) leak Hematoma (epidural, subdural, subarachnoid, intracerebral, intraventricular) Diffuse axonal injury Edema Traumatic brain injury Edema Concussion Foreign body	Recurrent CSF leak Meningitis Brain abscess
Nasolacrimal apparatus	Lacrimal injury	Epiphora Dacrocystitis
Parotid gland	Hematoma Infection Sialocele Salivary fistula Abscess	Sialocele Salivary fistula Parotitis Chronic pain Frey syndrome Facial deformity
Eye	Traumatic optic neuropathy Retrobulbar hematoma Globe rupture Vision loss Diplopia Muscle entrapment Enophthalmos Corneal abrasion Superior orbital fissure syndrome Orbital emphysema Oculocardiac reflex (bradycardia) Blindness Sympathetic ophthalmia	Persistent diplopia Enophthalmos Exopthalmos Lower-lid malposition Exposure keratitis Blindness Sympathetic ophthalmia
Bone	Fracture Bone loss	Delayed union Nonunion Malunion Infection/osteomyelitis
Dentition	Malocclusion Direct injury to tooth root Avulsion	Malocclusion Tooth loss Infection/abscess

headaches, or recurrent meningitis, and can be confirmed with a positive β2-transferrin test of collected fluid.[4] Most CSF leaks resulting from accidental and surgical trauma heal with conservative measures over the course of 7 to 10 days, although waiting for the leak to close spontaneously can increase the risk of meningitis, and close assessment to assure that complete resolution has occurred is necessary.[6] Surgical management includes exposure of the leak with primary repair or patch placement. Meningitis is treated aggressively with parenteral broad-spectrum antibiotics.

To prevent irreversible neurologic injury, spinal-cord injury should be suspected in all trauma patients until it is ruled out. Repair of facial fractures may initially be delayed while the patient is hemodynamically stabilized. If repair is performed before clearance of the cervical spine, it is imperative that the cervical spine remains in a neutral position. Closed reduction or external fixation techniques may be necessary to avoid injury to the spinal cord if access is inadequate.

Approximately 22% to 30% of orbital fractures have associated ocular injuries.[7] It is imperative

Table 2
Complications of facial trauma: upper, middle, and lower face

	Early	Late/Postoperative
Skull fracture	Traumatic brain injury Meningitis/brain abscess CSF leak Pneumocephalus Traumatic optic neuropathy Retrobulbar hematoma Cranial nerve injuries	Recurrent CSF Anosmia Meningitis/brain abscess Seizure Chronic sinusitis Cavernous sinus thrombosis Blindness Subdural hematoma
Frontal sinus fracture	CSF leak Traumatic brain injury Meningitis Pneumocephalus	Chronic sinusitis Alopecia Mucocele/mucopyocele Meningitis/brain abscess Osteomyelitis Encephalocele Frontal neuralgia Forehead deformity
ZMC fracture	Facial deformity Orbital injury Malocclusion Enophthalmos	Enophthalmos Facial deformity Diplopia Malar flattening Canthal malposition Ectropion
NOE fracture	CSF leak Telecanthus Chronic sinusitis Enophthalmos Anosmia Ocular Injury Traumatic brain injury	Telecanthus Persistent nasal deformity Pseudohypertelorism Scarring Forehead paresthesia Enophthalmos Diplopia Epiphora Dacrocystitis Anosmia Midface retrusion
Orbital fracture	Diplopia Enophthalmos Entrapment Cheek numbness (CN V2) Traumatic optic neuropathy Globe rupture Retrobulbar hematoma Oculocardiac reflex (bradycardia) Corneal abrasion Exopthalmos Lacrimal duct injury	Scleral show/lower-lid retraction Persistent diplopia Ectropion/entropion Enophthalmos Persistent entrapment Prominent scar Lower-lid edema Cheek numbness (CN V2) Canthal malposition Corneal abrasion Ptosis Epiphora Exposure keratitis Blindness Telecanthus Vertical dystopia
Nasal fracture	Septal hematoma Deviated nasal dorsum Nasal obstruction Epistaxis	Deviated septum Nasal obstruction Nasal deformity Septal perforation

(continued on next page)

Table 2 (continued)		
	Early	**Late/Postoperative**
Mandible	Malocclusion Facial paresthesia (CN V2, 3) Trismus Facial deformity Airway compromise Dental injury	Malocclusion Facial paralysis (CN V2, V3) Trismus Facial deformity Hardware exposure Dental injury Delayed union Nonunion Infection/osteomyelitis Malunion TMJ ankylosis

Abbreviations: CN, cranial nerve; CSF, cerebrospinal fluid; NOE, nasoorbitoethmoid; TMJ, temporomandibular joint; ZMC, zygomaticomaxillary complex.

that all patients are evaluated for vision-threatening injuries and managed emergently to minimize loss of vision (**Table 4**). The most common vision-threatening injuries include traumatic optic neuropathy, retrobulbar hemorrhage, and penetrating globe injury.[8] Visual acuity, visual fields, color vision, extraocular movement, the pupil, and the fundus should be examined in all patients with periorbital injuries. Diplopia, caused by inflammation and/or edema, is common after both orbital injury and surgery. It may also be evidence of direct injury to the globe, entrapment of orbital soft tissue or extraocular muscles, and vascular or neural damage. Diplopia is usually temporary and should be closely monitored. If persistent after surgical repair, a computed tomography (CT) scan should be obtained to evaluate the implant and fracture repair for misplacement and/or incarceration of soft tissue.[9] Unless entrapment or adherence has been identified, surgical exploration is rarely beneficial, and strabismus surgery may be required.[7,9,10] The presence of a retinal injury may preclude immediate repair of periorbital bone injuries, and surgery should be delayed until approved by the consultant ophthalmologist.

Soft-tissue injuries inferior to a line from the tragus to the upper lip should be evaluated for parotid injury. Penetrating injuries anterior to the posterior border of the masseter muscle require surgical exploration to evaluate for ductal injury. Sialoceles and salivary fistulas are managed conservatively, with surgery reserved for recalcitrant cases.[11] If a facial paralysis is present, wounds proximal to the lateral canthus and the nasolabial fold should be explored for facial nerve injury, and the nerve should be immediately repaired (**Table 5**).[12]

UPPER THIRD OF FACE

Fractures of the anterior skull base and frontal sinuses often are associated with traumatic brain injury, ocular injury, and CSF leak. Fractures of the anterior skull base can cause a tear in the underlying dura with subsequent CSF leak and risk for meningitis. Persistent CSF leak or a penetrating brain injury, such as displaced bone fragments, will require surgical intervention with either a transcranial approach or an endoscopic or subcranial extracranial approach. When the frontal sinus is fractured, multiple treatment options exist depending on the severity of the anterior table fracture, involvement of the frontal sinus outflow tract, and displacement of the posterior table. Most complications occur secondarily to inadequate removal of the mucosal lining after a frontal sinus obliteration or cranialization procedure, or are due to a failure to recognize compromise of the frontal sinus outflow tract(s) (FSOT). Long-term follow-up with CT evaluation is needed to monitor for insidious mucocele or encephalocele formation. With the advances of endoscopic sinus surgery, damage to the FSOT can often be managed expectantly with close observation and routine endoscopic evaluation, particularly when there is no involvement of the posterior wall. Delayed complications may be managed using the techniques of endoscopic sinus surgery.

MIDDLE THIRD OF THE FACE
Periorbital Complications

Most complications in the periorbital region are secondary to soft-tissue damage during surgical repair, improper placement of orbital implants, and inadequate reduction of the 3-dimensionally complex zygomaticomaxillary fracture (**Table 6**).

Table 3
Intracranial complications

Traumatic brain injury (TBI)	Closed head TBI	Typically a result of blunt impact. May result in a focal lesion in the brain (hematoma) or diffuse axonal injury (from shearing of axons against the skull base)	Neurosurgical consultation necessary
	Penetrating TBI	Occurs with foreign body violation of the skull and dura, entering the brain parenchyma. The size, speed, and track of the projectile determine the extent of neurologic damage	Neurosurgical consultation necessary
	Explosive blast TBI	More common in military combat and causes diffuse injury secondary to a pressure wave. Often results in rapidly developing cerebral edema, subarachnoid hemorrhage, and burst-pattern skull fractures	Neurosurgical consultation necessary
Cerebrospinal fluid (CSF) leak	Symptoms: persistent clear rhinorrhea or otorrhea, description of salty taste in mouth, headaches or recurrent meningitis	Neurosurgical or otolaryngology consultation may be necessary. Conservative management: bed rest, head elevation, avoidance of nose blowing or straining, and stool softeners. Antibiotic prophylaxis and lumbar drain placement is controversial and often surgeon dependent. Current studies have found no benefit from prophylactic antibiotics, though remains controversial[31] Surgical management: transcranial, subcranial, or endoscopic approach with the placement of a mucosal, fascial, or bone graft.[4] The endoscopic approach has become more prevalent and is shown to be safe and effective, with a 90% initial success rate that improves further with subsequent attempts, with lower morbidities than open procedures[32]	
Meningitis	Symptoms: headache, nausea, photophobia, altered level of consciousness, fever, nuchal rigidity and pain with flexion of the neck	Empiric first-line treatment in patients with postneurosurgical meningitis is intravenous vancomycin plus cefepime or ceftazidime[33]	

Table 4
Ocular complications

Retrobulbar hematoma (RBH)	Bleeding into the orbit causing increased intraocular pressure compromising the blood supply to the optic nerve and retina. Leads to progressive vision loss and eventual blindness Venous: Slower progression. May not be evident until patient is in recovery or possibly after discharge Arterial: Can progress within seconds, requiring frequent monitoring or palpation of the globe during surgery, especially if significant bleeding is encountered	Symptoms: proptosis, periorbital ecchymosis, increased intraocular pressure, tense globe, loss of direct pupillary light reflex, diplopia, ophthalmoplegia, and decreasing visual acuity/blindness	*First-line treatment:* Immediate lateral canthotomy and inferior cantholysis *Adjunctive treatment:* Head of bed elevation or reverse Trendelenburg (cervical-spine precautions), removal of intranasal packing, and immediate ophthalmology consultation with measurement of intraocular pressure. Administration of mannitol 20% (1–2 g/kg IV over 30–60 min), systemic corticosteroids (dexamethasone 8–10 mg IV every 8 h for 3–4 doses), acetazolamide (500 mg IV bolus) or topical antiglaucoma eye drops (Timolol ophthalmic drops 0.5%, 1–2 drops topically twice daily)[10,34] *Second-line treatment:* Orbital decompression and anterior/posterior ethmoid artery ligation
Traumatic optic neuropathy (TON)	Clinical diagnosis referring to any insult to the optic nerve secondary to trauma Direct TON: penetrating injuries severing the optic nerve. Permanent blindness results Indirect TON: hematoma or secondary edema of the optic nerve within optic canal causing direct mechanical trauma or vascular ischemia, leading to further retinal ganglion cell injury and visual loss	Symptoms: relative afferent pupillary defect in the affected eye and varying loss of visual acuity from partial visual loss to blindness	Ophthalmology consultation is necessary *Treatment:* No standard of care. Options include observation, corticosteroids, and optic nerve decompression. Spontaneous visual recovery ranges from 0% to 60%. At present neither intervention has been found to be more effective than observation alone. Patients presenting with no perception of light to the injured eye have a poor prognosis for recovery with any course of action[8]

(continued on next page)

Table 4
(continued)

Open globe injury/globe rupture	Full-thickness defect of the cornea or sclera	Findings: possible prolapsing uveal tissue, retina, or vitreous gel. Decreased intraocular pressure	Do not manipulate the eye to prevent extrusion of contents. A protective eye shield is placed and emergent ophthalmology consultation is made. Early surgical repair, if possible. Enucleation or evisceration of the globe within 2 weeks with nonsalvageable injuries to avoid sympathetic ophthalmia[8]
Sympathetic ophthalmia	Rare, bilateral, granulomatous uveitis presenting after ocular trauma or surgical interventions, causing blindness in the noninjured (sympathetic) eye. Etiology thought to involve inflammatory and autoimmune response after ocular antigens exposed to the immune system. Presents weeks to years after injury	Symptoms: insidious onset of blurry vision, pain, epiphora, and photophobia	Ophthalmology consultation is necessary. Aggressive treatment with systemic corticosteroids or immunosuppressive therapy[35]

Abbreviation: IV, intravenous.

Lower-lid malposition

Lower-lid malpositions include scleral show, lower-lid retraction, ectropion, and entropion.[13] Although mild cases may resolve with conservative measures, persistent malposition can lead to significant morbidity. Close attention to surgical technique and retraction of periorbital soft tissue may help prevent lid malpositions after surgical treatment. Patients at increased risk for malposition may benefit from the addition of canthopexy, canthoplasty, lateral tarsal strip procedure, or resuspension of the orbicularis oculi and/or suborbicularis oculi fat at the time of repair. A temporary Frost suspension suture or tarsorrhaphy can help prevent vertical contracture during the early healing phase.[13,14] An ectropion is an outward rotation of the eyelid margin and is most common with the subciliary lower-eyelid approach.[7,13,14] Ectropion is caused by laxity of the canthal tendons and orbicularis oculi, disinsertion of the lower-lid retractors, or vertical contracture of anterior lamella after trauma or surgery.[14] Surgical treatment

involves correction of the horizontal laxity with a tightening procedure, release of the scar, and a full-thickness skin graft. Entropion is defined as an inward rotation of the eyelid margin, and often results in significant ocular discomfort owing to chronic irritation from the eyelashes (trichiasis). This condition is secondary to contracture of the posterior lamella of the eyelid and canthal laxity. Although the risk is low, it is increased when the transconjunctival approach is used.[13] Repair may be performed with repositioning sutures, but often requires lengthening of the posterior lamella with a graft and possible shortening of the anterior lamella.[14]

Entrapment

Entrapment occurs when the periorbital soft tissue herniates outside the orbit and becomes tethered on bony fragments or implants. It is most common in orbital-floor fractures but can occur anywhere along the periphery of the orbit. Entrapment causes dysmotility of the globe with subsequent

Table 5
Visceral complications

Lacrimal duct injury	Treatment: Ophthalmology consultation should be obtained. Primary repair and stent placement. Open or endoscopic dacrocystorhinostomy if lacrimal duct obstruction occurs[36]
Parotid duct injury	Treatment: A lacrimal probe is used to cannulate the duct through the papilla (opposite the second molar). If an injury is found, a tension-free primary repair over a silastic catheter with 9-0 nylon is performed. If it cannot be repaired primarily, proximal segment can be ligated or the distal end can be reimplanted into the buccal mucosa
Facial nerve injury	Treatment: Primary anastomosis with epineural 10-0 nylon if not under tension, otherwise an interposition graft (great auricular nerve) placed[12]

diplopia, and the herniation of soft tissue may contribute to enophthalmos. Gross entrapment may be assessed on examination of voluntary eye movement; however, definitive testing is performed using forced duction testing. It is imperative that after any orbital fracture repair, a forced duction test is performed to confirm adequate reduction of entrapped soft tissue and to ensure that inadvertent entrapment has not occurred.

Enophthalmos

Enophthalmos is posterior displacement of the globe secondary to increased orbital volume (most common) or loss of orbital soft tissue (less common) when the orbital floor and/or walls were not repaired or inadequate repair was performed. It is a common posttraumatic facial deformity that is often challenging to correct, particularly when scarring of the orbital soft tissues has developed.[7,15] Improper placement of an orbital implant and incomplete reduction of a zygomaticomaxillary complex (ZMC) fracture are common causes. For orbital-floor fractures, failure most often occurs from inadequate dissection and visualization of the posterior ledge of the orbital floor. This shortcoming may be due to a failure to

fully appreciate the posterosuperior angulation of the orbital floor from the anterior orbital rim and fear of injury to the optic nerve.[7,15] Endoscopically guided or assisted repair is helpful, as this technique increases posterior visualization via the maxillary sinus to ensure complete reduction of herniated soft tissue and proper implant placement. Surgical correction typically requires revision of an inadequately reduced ZMC fracture or improperly placed implant. More advanced surgical interventions may be required to adequately restore orbital volume, and computerized planning can sometimes be helpful in this situation.[16]

Zygomaticomaxillary Complex Fractures

ZMC fractures can cause significant impairment to function and appearance of the midface and orbit. It is the second most common facial fracture, and it is often a challenge to adequately repair these fractures with a high potential for complications.[17] The ZMC is an important buttress for the face, provides the prominence of the cheek, and determines the midface width with the zygomatic arch. Fractures may be isolated or comminuted, and proper diagnosis, precise reduction, and adequate fixation are keys for successful repair. Inadequate reduction produces malar flattening, increased facial width, and external rotation of the lateral orbital walls, resulting in enophthalmos.[15] When significant postoperative asymmetry exists, osteotomies and bone grafting may be required.

Nasal Fractures

The nasal bones are the most commonly fractured facial bones. Epistaxis should be controlled and septal hematomas should be immediately drained. Displaced nasal fractures are typically treated with closed reduction in the acute setting (within the first 14 days). A formal septorhinoplasty is typically reserved for continued deformity or nasal obstruction 6 to 9 months after the initial injury, allowing for adequate healing.[18]

Nasoorbitoethmoid Fractures

Nasoorbitoethmoid (NOE) fractures can be extremely challenging to properly repair. Inadequate repair often results in secondary deformities that are even more difficult and, at times, impossible to reconstruct.[19] The most common long-term complications include telecanthus (lateral displacement of the medial canthal ligament(s), which gives the appearance of hypertelorism, and is therefore also called pseudohypertelorism) and dorsal nasal collapse.[20,21] Reconstruction requires reduction and stabilization of the central fragment and medial canthal tendon, often requiring bone

Table 6
Eyelid and periorbital complications

Complication	Description	Management
Lower eyelid retraction	Eyelid margin is inferiorly displaced with respect to its natural resting position against the cornea. Typically occurs in combination with an ectropion or entropion	Initial management: Massage, artificial tears, lubricating ointment, and eye taping Surgical management: Lateral canthal tightening procedure
Ectropion	Outward rotation of the eyelid margin Involutional ectropion: Laxity of the medial and lateral canthal tendons, disinsertion of the lower-lid retractors, or atrophy of the orbicularis muscle Paralytic ectropion: Deinnervation of the orbicularis oculi muscle after trauma to facial nerve Cicatricial ectropion: Vertical contracture of the skin and/or orbicularis oculi muscle (anterior lamella)	Initial management: Massage, artificial tears, lubricating ointment, and eye taping Surgical management: Lateral canthal tightening procedure for horizontal laxity. Cicatricial ectropion also requires release of contracture and full-thickness skin graft from the upper eyelid, postauricular or supraclavicular region to prevent repeat scar contraction and restore tissue deficiency of the anterior lamella, and restore tissue deficiency of the anterior lamella
Entropion	Inward rotation of the eyelid margin Cicatricial entropion: contracture of the conjunctiva and tarsal plate (posterior lamella) of the eyelid	Initial management: Massage, artificial tears, lubricating ointment, and eye taping Conservative treatment: Placement of Quickert-Rathbun full-thickness rotation sutures to evert the lid[14] Surgical treatment: Scar excision and graft placement to lengthen the posterior lamella. Graft choices include buccal, hard palate or nasal mucosa, upper eyelid tarsus, or conchal cartilage. Lateral canthal tightening for horizontal laxity
Enophthalmos	Posterior displacement of the globe secondary to increased orbital volume	Etiology determined by computed tomography scan Remobilization of inadequately reduced ZMC fracture with anatomic reduction and fixation. Osteotomies and bone grafts may be required Orbital floor or medial orbital wall repair with implant placement. If improperly placed implant already in place, remove and replace in anatomic position. If significant scarring is present at the interface between the implant and periorbita (titanium mesh implant), the implant can be elevated with the periorbita and a second implant placed underneath.[7] Additional grafting or implants may be required to restore orbital volume. The use of computerized planning and intraoperative navigational guidance are new tools, which may assist in proper positioning of implants and improved outcomes Perform forced duction test at end of procedure to ensure entrapment of soft tissue has not occurred[7]
Telecanthus	Increased distance between medial canthi of the eyelids	Treatment: Transnasal wiring procedure with recreation of normal intercanthal distance (equal to the width of the alar base or half the interpupillary distance)

grafts and transnasal wire fixation. Severe fractures will result in significant loss of nasal support and projection, requiring a cantilevered bone graft and columellar strut graft to restore adequate height, length, and projection. Soft-tissue contraction can make delayed nasal reconstruction less successful, so it is best to obtain proper nasal positioning during primary repair.[22]

LOWER THIRD OF THE FACE
Mandible

The goals of mandibular fracture repair are to produce pain-free mobility of the jaw with adequate mouth opening, restoration of premorbid occlusion, good facial and jaw symmetry, osseous union of fractures, and return to baseline functioning.[23] Malocclusion, infection, and abnormal bone healing are common complications of mandibular trauma, and are often due to incompletely reduced or inadequately fixated fractures (**Table 7**). The increased use of open reduction with internal fixation techniques has allowed for quicker return to functional recovery. This concept, however, requires precise anatomic reduction of fractured segments and stable fixation to maintain correct position against mechanical forces produced by motion.[24] Infection after fracture repair is typically due to inadequate fixation or technical errors in hardware placement. Any motion across the fracture or screws holding the reduction will result in resorption of bone, often leading to further instability, infection, extrusion, and, potentially, nonunion.[25] Other risk factors for infection include a delay in treatment, previous infection, poor surgical technique, dental abnormality, poor patient compliance, drug and alcohol abuse, operative experience of the surgeon, and severity of fracture(s).[26] Soft-tissue infections are managed with drainage and culture-directed antibiotic therapy without removal of hardware as long as the fixation is stable and the screws are tight. Loose screws should prompt wound exploration and hardware removal, and stronger (usually load-bearing) fixation should be reapplied if the fracture is still mobile.[24] If a chronic infection with osteomyelitis is determined radiographically and/or clinically, the patient is treated with open reduction, debridement of infected/necrotic bone, and placement of a mandibular reconstruction plate.[27] Immediate or delayed bone grafts are used if there is inadequate bone stock. Patients are then followed while being treated with prolonged culture-directed antibiotic therapy. Restoration of premorbid occlusion is one of the key goals of fracture treatment and serves as a reference for premorbid skeletal position. Malocclusion results when rigid fixation is performed with the bones in an improper position. Approximation of wear facets and discussion with the patient or family will guide the treatment of patients with abnormal premorbid occlusion.

MANAGEMENT
Preoperative

The advanced traumatic life-support protocol should be performed with emergent airway intervention and control of hemorrhage. Once stabilized, a thorough history and physical examination with documentation of mental status, cranial nerve examination, ocular examination, and occlusion should be obtained, along with photographic documentation of all facial injuries. High-resolution CT imaging (1-mm thick sections with multiplanar reconstructions) with axial, coronal, and sagittal views allows for optimal visualization of fracture patterns. For complex facial fractures, 3-dimensional reconstruction CT scans can be helpful in planning an operative strategy. Mandible fractures should have a panorex image, if the patient is capable. Appropriate consultation with neurosurgery, ophthalmology, and other appropriate services should be made for treatment planning and coordination of management. Timing of repair depends on multiple factors; however, successful fracture repair is best achieved as early as possible. Complex trauma is often delayed a few days because of the presence of other more life-threatening injuries. Delay in repair leads to increased bacterial contamination, infection, callus formation, and soft-tissue fibrosis and contraction, making mobility and accurate reduction more difficult to achieve.[24] Antibiotic therapy should be initiated on grossly infected wounds, facial fractures, and mandibular fractures.

Perioperative/Intraoperative

Perioperative intravenous antibiotics should be given before the start of the operation. Recent advances in intraoperative imaging may assist in avoiding complications during the procedure. Intraoperative CT imaging can confirm adequate reduction of complex fractures and proper placement of orbital implants, allowing for repositioning before completion of the procedure. Image-guidance systems have been a useful tool for endoscopic procedures near the skull base, and 3-dimensional computer-based algorithms may assist with treatment planning.[15,28]

Postoperative

Examination of visual acuity and the facial nerves should be performed in the recovery area, with

Table 7 Common complications of mandibular fractures	
Delayed union	Reduced or absent mineralization of a fracture 8–12 wk after immobilization. Treatment includes continued observation and prolonged interdental fixation. Classic description, but not really relevant in the age of rigid fixation
Nonunion	Failure to progress to ossification during indirect healing. Typically involves a wider segment with poor functional results. Patients typically develop pain, trismus, and infection. Must treat the infection, remobilize fragments with removal of callus/granulation tissue, and repeat reduction and fixation
Malunion	Fracture heals by osseous union with segments in nonanatomic position. Requires remobilization of involved bones with osteotomies followed by repositioning and fixation in proper occlusion. Bone grafts may be needed in areas of bone loss
Symphysis	In the symphyseal region torsional forces are present in addition to tension and compression forces. Two points of fixation are required to resist the torsional force. Careful attention must be given to potential widening of the mandible because of lingual splaying of the symphyseal fracture
Body	Care must be taken to avoid damage to the inferior alveolar nerve and tooth roots with screw placement
Angle	Adequate fixation of noncomminuted angle fractures is controversial with regard to 1- or 2-plate fixation. Recent literature has shown a decreased risk of complications and shorter operative time with a single miniplate at the oblique line, although Fox and Kellman have demonstrated better results using 2 miniplates.[37,38] In a comminuted angle fracture a load-bearing reconstruction bar is required
Condyle	Can be treated successfully with closed management or open reduction and internal fixation (ORIF). Relative indications for ORIF include bilateral condylar fractures to restore lower facial height, concomitant comminuted maxillary fractures, edentulous patients for immediate return of function and ability to wear dentures, those who cannot tolerate or do not want prolonged use of arch bars and elastics, or do not want the cosmetic deformity that occurs with foreshortening the side of the fracture. Closed management requires a good complement of teeth, especially posteriorly to maintain posterior vertical height. The patient must be cooperative with posttreatment elastics for 4–6 wk, functional exercises, and close follow-up. Relative indications for closed management: when precise reduction and internal fixation cannot be obtained, other life-threatening injuries and shorter anesthetic time is indicated, intracapsular condylar fractures, or in cervical spine precautions with limited access
Atrophic mandible	Requires a large load-bearing mandibular reconstruction plate, may require bone graft
Tooth in fracture line	The decision to retain or remove a tooth in a fracture line is controversial, and occurs most commonly with third molars. There is concern for increased risk of infection and nonunion; however, extraction may add additional trauma to the adjacent bone and destabilize the fracture. It is generally accepted that healthy third molars not interfering with fracture reduction should be retained. Extraction is indicated for significant caries, mobility, a tooth preventing reduction of the fracture, fractured or exposed roots, or a recurring abscess at the fracture site despite antibiotic therapy

serial ocular examination if indicated. Prophylactic antibiotics should be continued up to 24 hours after surgery, with further use at the discretion of the surgeon; however, current literature has not shown benefit of prolonged prophylactic antibiotics.[29] If an intraoperative CT scan was not performed, a postoperative CT scan is useful to evaluate placement of orbital implants and the position of the fixated fractures. Patient compliance is difficult to control and can have a significant impact on postoperative complications. Counseling and education should be performed to encourage long-term follow-up. Mandibular fractures treated with guiding elastics should be followed closely for functional rehabilitation and maintenance of occlusion.

PHARMACOLOGIC COMPLICATIONS

There is little discussion in the literature regarding pharmacologic interventions that may contribute to facial trauma complications. It should be noted that patients on anticoagulation or antiplatelet therapy have an increased risk for hematoma, which can be detrimental in orbital or skull-base surgery.[30] Surgeons should closely monitor these patients in the postoperative period, with a low threshold on intervention. The use of adrenaline or local anesthetic with epinephrine near the eye can result in transient pupillary dilation, which can create anxiety for the surgeon and should be monitored until it has fully resolved.

SUMMARY

Management of facial trauma can be very challenging for the surgeon, who of course desires to obtain the best possible outcome. Adequate preoperative planning, including appropriate consultations and sometimes computerized planning, can help ensure the best possible results. Once in surgery, intraoperative CT and navigation can assist with this as well. Careful assessment postoperatively will allow early recognition of less than favorable results, and a willingness to reoperate in such situations will also lead to better long-term outcomes.

REFERENCES

1. Leach J. Proper handling of soft tissue in the acute phase. Facial Plast Surg 2001;17(4):227–38.
2. Mulligan RP, Mahabir RC. The prevalence of cervical spine injury, head injury, or both with isolated and multiple craniomaxillofacial fractures. Plast Reconstr Surg 2010;126:1647–51.
3. Ling GS, Ecklund JM. Traumatic brain injury in modern war. Curr Opin Anaesthesiol 2011;24(2):124–30.
4. Kerr JT, Chu FW, Bayles SW. Cerebrospinal fluid rhinorrhea: diagnosis and management. Otolaryngol Clin North Am 2005;38(4):597–611.
5. Friedman JA, Ebersold MJ, Quast LM. Post-traumatic cerebrospinal fluid leakage. World J Surg 2001;25(8):1062–6.
6. Martin TJ, Loehrl TA. Endoscopic CSF leak repair. Curr Opin Otolaryngol Head Neck Surg 2007; 15(1):35–9.
7. Cole P, Kaufman Y, Hollier L. Principles of facial trauma: orbital fracture management. J Craniofac Surg 2009;20(1):101–4.
8. McClenaghan FC, Ezra DG, Holmes SB. Mechanisms and management of vision loss following

9. Silbert DI, Matta NS, Singman EL. Diplopia secondary to orbital surgery. Am Orthopt J 2012;62: 22–8.
10. Silva AB, Stankiewicz JA. Perioperative and postoperative management of orbital complications in functional endoscopic sinus surgery. Oper Tech Otolaryngol Head Neck Surg 1995;6(3):231–6.
11. Gordin EA, Daniero JJ, Krein H, et al. Parotid gland trauma. Facial Plast Surg 2010;26(6):504–10.
12. Angeli SI, Chiossone E. Surgical treatment of the facial nerve in facial paralysis. Otolaryngol Clin North Am 1997;30(5):683–700.
13. Ridgway EB, Chen C, Colakoglu S, et al. The incidence of lower eyelid malposition after facial fracture repair: a retrospective study and meta-analysis comparing subtarsal, subciliary, and transconjunctival incisions. Plast Reconstr Surg 2009;124(5): 1578–86.
14. Vallabhanath P, Carter SR. Ectropion and entropion. Curr Opin Ophthalmol 2000;11(5):345–51.
15. Chen CT, Huang F, Chen YR. Management of posttraumatic enophthalmos. Chang Gung Med J 2006;29(3):251–61.
16. Bly RA, Chang SH, Cudejkova M, et al. Computer-guided orbital reconstruction to improve outcomes. JAMA Facial Plast Surg 2013;15(2):113–20.
17. Lee EI, Mohan K, Koshy JC, et al. Optimizing the surgical management of zygomaticomaxillary complex fractures. Semin Plast Surg 2010;24(4):389–97.
18. Chan J, Most SP. Diagnosis and management of nasal fractures. Oper Tech Otolaryngol Head Neck Surg 2008;19(4):263–6.
19. Schaller B. Subcranial approach in the surgical treatment of anterior skull base trauma. Acta Neurochir (Wien) 2005;147(4):355–66.
20. O-Lee TJ, Koltai PJ. Pediatric orbital roof fractures. Oper Tech Otolaryngol Head Neck Surg 2008; 19(2):98–107.
21. Imola MJ, Ducic Y, Adelson RT. The secondary correction of post-traumatic craniofacial deformities. Otolaryngol Head Neck Surg 2008;139(5): 654–60.
22. Potter JK, Muzaffar AR, Ellis E, et al. Aesthetic management of the nasal component of naso-orbital ethmoid fractures. Plast Reconstr Surg 2006; 117(1):10e–8e.
23. Zachariades N, Mezitis M, Mourouzis C, et al. Fractures of the mandibular condyle: a review of 466 cases: literature review, reflections on treatment and proposals. J Craniomaxillofac Surg 2006; 34(7):421–32.
24. Kellman RM, Tatum SA. Complex facial trauma with plating. In: Bailey BJ, editor. Head and neck surgery—otolaryngology. 2nd edition. Philadelphia: Lippincott-Raven Publishers; 1998. p. 1043–60.

25. Shumrick KA. Complications of facial plating. Oper Tech Otolaryngol Head Neck Surg 1995; 6(2):135–41.

26. Kellman RM, Wright DL. Management of posttraumatic osteomyelitis of the mandible. Chapter 39. In: Greenberg AM, Prein J, editors. Craniomaxillofacial reconstructive and corrective bone surgery: principles of internal fixation using the AO/ASIF technique. New York: Springer-Verlag; 2002. p. 433–8.

27. Moreno JC, Fernandez A, Ortiz JA, et al. Complication rates associated with different treatments for mandibular fractures. J Oral Maxillofac Surg 2000; 58(3):273–80.

28. Essig H, Rana M, Kokemueller H, et al. Pre-operative planning for mandibular reconstruction—a full digital planning workflow resulting in a patient specific reconstruction. Head Neck Oncol 2011;3:45.

29. Abubaker AO, Rollert MK. Postoperative antibiotic prophylaxis in mandibular fractures: a preliminary randomized, double-blind, and placebo-controlled clinical study. J Oral Maxillofac Surg 2001;59(12): 1415–9.

30. Gosau M, Schöneich M, Draenert FG, et al. Retrospective analysis of orbital floor fractures—complications, outcome, and review of literature. Clin Oral Investig 2011;15(3):305–13.

31. Ratilal BO, Costa J, Sampaio C, et al. Antibiotic prophylaxis for preventing meningitis in patients with basilar skull fractures. Cochrane Database Syst Rev 2011;(8):CD004884.

32. Psaltis AJ, Schlosser RJ, Banks CA, et al. A systematic review of the endoscopic repair of cerebrospinal fluid leaks. Otolaryngol Head Neck Surg 2012;147(2):196–203.

33. van de Beek D, Brouwer MC, Thwaites GE, et al. Advances in treatment of bacterial meningitis. Lancet 2012;380(9854):1693–702.

34. Viterbo S, Boffano P, Guglielmi V, et al. Double consecutive retrobulbar hemorrhage in a high-risk patient in treatment with aspirin and warfarin. J Craniofac Surg 2012;23(6):1782–4.

35. Damico FM, Kiss S, Young LH. Sympathetic ophthalmia. Semin Ophthalmol 2005;20(3):191–7.

36. Ali MJ, Gupta H, Honavar SG, et al. Acquired nasolacrimal duct obstructions secondary to naso-orbito-ethmoidal fractures: patterns and outcomes. Ophthal Plast Reconstr Surg 2012;28(4):242–5.

37. Ellis E 3rd. A prospective study of 3 treatment methods for isolated fractures of the mandibular angle. J Oral Maxillofac Surg 2010;68(11):2743–54.

38. Fox AJ, Kellman RM. Mandibular angle fractures: two-miniplate fixation and complications. Arch Facial Plast Surg 2003;5:464–9.

Complications of Forehead Lift

Jessyka G. Lighthall, MD, Tom D. Wang, MD*

KEYWORDS

- Brow lift • Forehead lift • Complications in cosmetic surgery • Brow rejuvenation
- Forehead anatomy

KEY POINTS

- A thorough understanding of brow anatomy, patient variations, and potential complications is requisite for surgeons performing forehead rejuvenation.
- As with every aspect of facial plastic surgery, the prevention of postoperative patient dissatisfaction begins with a careful patient history inclusive of psychiatric history, motivation and expectations for surgery, and investment in the outcome.
- In-depth knowledge of a patient's medical history is important to identify patients who are poor surgical candidates and are at high risk of medical complications.
- Overall, complications can be minimized by a thorough preoperative history and physical examination combined with meticulous technique, conservative suspension, and a tension-free wound closure.

INTRODUCTION

Patients often present with the complaint of tired-appearing eyes with excessive eyelid skin. The astute aesthetic surgeon may note on examination the contribution of brow ptosis to the overall heavy appearance of the patient's upper eyelids with or without true dermatochalasis. Rejuvenation of the forehead may result in a more youthful appearance and may reduce or negate the necessity of blepharoplasty in some patients. A thorough understanding of the anatomy, patient variations, and potential complications is requisite for surgeons performing forehead rejuvenation.

FOREHEAD ANATOMY

Critical to facial rejuvenation is an understanding of the anatomy.

Brow Soft Tissue

In the forehead, the soft tissue layers include skin, subcutaneous tissue, muscle, fibrous galea, loose areolar tissue, and pericranium.[1] The superficial musculoaponeurotic system in the inferior two-thirds of the face continues over the zygoma as the superficial temporoparietal fascia, which merges with the galea in the forehead. The temporal line, which is formed by the convergence of the deep and superficial layers of the deep temporal fascia investing the temporalis muscle with the frontal periosteum, meets the lateral margin of the galea to form the conjoined tendon. Another important landmark in brow lifting procedures is the densely adherent arcus marginalis along the supraorbital rim, which is where the frontal periosteum fuses with the galea. Release of these dense fibrous attachments in forehead rejuvenation is vital to produce the desired elevation and stabilization of the brow.

Brow Muscles

The muscles important to brow surgery are the frontalis muscle, paired corrugator supercilii muscles, and procerus muscle.[2] The frontalis, which

Disclosures: None.
Department of Otolaryngology/Head and Neck Surgery, Oregon Health and Science University, Mailcode: SJH-01, 3181 Southwest Sam Jackson Park Road, Portland, OR 97239, USA
* Corresponding author.
E-mail address: wangt@ohsu.edu

Facial Plast Surg Clin N Am 21 (2013) 619–624
http://dx.doi.org/10.1016/j.fsc.2013.07.006
1064-7406/13/$ – see front matter © 2013 Elsevier Inc. All rights reserved.

has a natural dehiscence in the midline, is a thin, fan-like muscle that acts largely to elevate the brow. This muscle is responsible for the development of horizontal rhytids with age.

The paired corrugator supercilii muscles have two heads, including transversely oriented fibers along the medial supraorbital rim acting to pull the brows medially, and oblique fibers that act to depress the medial brow. The corrugator muscles cause the vertically oriented rhytids that develop in the glabellar region.

The procerus muscle runs vertically from the nasal bones to the frontalis muscle and depresses the medial brow. It is responsible for the transversely oriented rhytids in the region of the radix. The medial brow is also depressed by the medial fibers of the orbicular is oculi muscles. Superior fibers of the latter depress the brow along its length.

Brow Innervation

Sensory innervation to the lateral and central forehead come from branches of the trigeminal nerve and run to the vertex of the scalp with subgaleal extensions. The ophthalmic division of the trigeminal nerve gives off the supratrochlear and supraorbital branches, whereas the maxillary division provides temporal sensation by the auriculotemporal and zygomaticotemporal branches. Motor innervation to the forehead is by the temporal branch of the facial nerve. The main trunk of the facial nerve exits the stylomastoid foramen, divides within the parotid, and travels deep to the superficial musculoaponeurotic system, giving off its terminal branches. The temporal branch is located just superficial to the zygomatic arch periosteum in the middle third, approximately 1.5 cm lateral to the lateral orbital rim. From here, it continues in the temporoparietal fascia to enter the undersurface of the brow musculature approximately 1 cm above the supraorbital rim.[3] Appreciating and protecting the motor innervation is of the utmost importance during any approach to forehead lifting.

Brow Vasculature

There is a robust blood supply to the forehead from the internal and external carotid systems. Contributions of the internal carotid artery by the ophthalmic branch are the supratrocheal and supraorbital bundle, which travel with similarly names sensory nerves. These neurovascular bundles are found deep to the frontalis muscle until approximately 1 cm above the supraorbital rim when they pierce this muscle to run more superficially. The remainder of the blood supply can be found in the subcutaneous plane. The location of

the vascular supply should be considered when deciding on a given approach to forehead lifting. Key venous anatomy is the sentinel vein, which runs superficial to the deep temporal fascia near the region of the frontozygomatic suture. Identification of this vein, particularly in endoscopic approaches, assists the surgeon in locating and avoiding the temporal branch of the facial nerve as it runs in close approximation and superficial to this vessel.[4] In addition, the sentinel vein can pose a significant bleeding problem if not properly identified and preserved or cauterized.

PREVENTION OF COMPLICATIONS IN BROW SURGERY
Patient History

As with every aspect of facial plastic surgery, the prevention of postoperative patient dissatisfaction begins with a careful patient history inclusive of psychiatric history, motivation and expectations for surgery, and investment in the outcome.[5] The presence of body dysmorphic disorder should be identified preoperatively and cosmetic surgical procedures in this patient group should be avoided. History of prior surgery should be elucidated. Concurrent desire for upper and/or lower eyelid rejuvenation should be discussed, and an ocular history taken to determine the presence of vision loss, dry eye syndrome, use of lubricating ophthalmic drops, or prior ocular surgery.[6] Often, the symptoms may be subtle and include burning of eyes or a foreign body sensation. This history is key for avoidance of postoperative ocular complications.

In-depth knowledge of a patient's medical history is important to identify patients who are poor surgical candidates and are at high risk of medical complications. Elective operations in high-risk patients should be carefully considered. Any personal or family history of coagulopathies should be noted, as should a personal history of a bleeding complication after prior surgery. An evaluation for bleeding disorders should be completed in these patients. Patients should be informed to avoid blood thinners and herbal supplements with blood-thinning properties.

Physical Examination

A thorough physical examination is requisite and knowledge of ideal brow position is vital. The distance from the midpupil to the upper edge of the eyebrow is 2.5 cm.[7] The ideal brow position in females is considered to be above the supraorbital rim with a gentle arc and a peak located over the lateral limbus.[7,8] The feminine brow is typically thicker medially and tapers laterally. For males, brow position is generally more horizontal, located at the supraorbital rim, and thicker. The presence of orbital and brow asymmetries should be noted, photographed, and discussed with the patient preoperatively.

A careful examination of the upper and lower eyelids should also be performed to identify dermatochalasis and blepharoptosis, which if not addressed concurrently may produce dissatisfaction in the postoperative forehead rejuvenation patient. Ptosis may be defined as palpebral fissure width measured at the central lid of less than 10 mm. Another method of assessing for ptosis is with the margin reflex distance-1, which measures the distance from the pupillary reflex to the central upper eyelid margin. Distances less than 4 mm may signify ptosis.[8]

In addition to the patient history, the examination should assess for signs of dry eye syndrome, including a roughened or irritated cornea, mucoid deposition along the lid margin, and signs of chronic irritation.[6] If there is any concern for dry eye syndrome, one should consider preoperative ophthalmologic evaluation and a Schirmer or tear breakup test should be performed. These symptoms may be exacerbated by periorbital surgery and forehead lifting.[6,9]

Finally, the complete examination should include an assessment of skin type, photoaging status, presence of hair loss or thinning, location of the hairline, and presence of static and dynamic glabellar and forehead rhytids. The ideal hairline is approximately 5 cm from the upper edge of the brow.[10] The length of the forehead and height of the hairline may influence the approach selected for rejuvenation.

TYPES OF FOREHEAD LIFT

Various types of forehead lift exist, and type chosen depends on surgeon and patient preference and patient characteristics. Knowledge of all techniques and ideal situations to use each technique is important to proper patient selection and good outcomes.

Direct Brow Lift

The direct brow lift involves an incision superior to the brow with excision of a variable amount of epidermis and dermis and includes suspension of the orbicularis oculi muscle to the pericranium. This approach is useful for unilateral facial paralysis and brow asymmetries, and is often used in men with thick eyebrows. Complications of this approach include persistent asymmetries, an unsightly scar, and anesthesia if the sensory nerves are disrupted by dissecting in the submuscular

plane. Another limitation of this approach is an inability to address the aging changes of the remainder of the forehead, which may limit the overall aesthetic outcome. However, in the properly selected patient, excellent results may be noted. This approach may also remove the fine vellus hairs above the brows, resulting in a "tweezed" appearance. This may result in feminizing a male brow and needs to be used with caution in male patients.

Midforehead Lift

Similarly, the midforehead approach is typically limited to men with deep forehead rhytids and male pattern baldness with brow ptosis but minimal concern for the remainder of the forehead. This approach involves an incision in an existing rhytid with skin excision. It carries the risk of a poor scar outcome and requires a meticulous, tension-free closure. As opposed to the direct brow lift, the midforehead lift allows the surgeon to address bilateral brow lines and involves orbicularis suspension. Some brow asymmetries may be addressed, although for large asymmetries, a unilateral direct approach may still be warranted. The risk of anesthesia also exists but may be minimized by dissection in the subdermal plane.

Coronal Lift

For many years, the workhorse approach for forehead lift was the coronal approach. Modifications include the trichophytic and pretrichophytic incision placement and dissection in various planes. This approach is well-suited for patients with a normal to low hairline and is traditionally contraindicated in patients with a high hairline or male pattern baldness because skin excision anterior to the incision raises the frontal hairline. Although it involves extensive dissection, this approach allows for excellent direct visualization of the forehead anatomy. The corrugator supercilii, the procerus, and the frontalis muscle may be easily addressed by myotomies or excision to limit postoperative muscle action, which may cause future static and dynamic rhytid formation. The galea is typically suspended to some degree, although a lift caused by skin excision alone may be performed. The extent of dissection theoretically increases the risk of adverse effects, which include elevation of the hairline, alopecia, presence of a prominent scar, hematoma formation, anesthesia, damage to the temporal branch of the facial nerve, and over elevation of the brow producing temporary or permanent lagophthalmos. The risk of the latter complication is heightened when a concomitant blepharoplasty is performed. Brow lift should always be performed first.

Multiple variations on the traditional coronal lift have been used to decrease complications and improve aesthetic outcomes. The trichophytic lift was designed to minimize elevation of the hair line or even assist with decreasing the height of the forehead in appropriately selected patients. One unique potential adverse effect is overshortening of the forehead with an aggressive skin excision or a larger area of postoperative anesthesia. The pretrichophytic modification is similarly indicated for patients with a long forehead or high hairline. The potential for a poor, visible scar is decreased by incision beveling, preserving skin appendages, and using a geometric broken line when making incisions. These modifications otherwise have similar potential complications as the traditional coronal technique. In each approach, the risks are minimized by meticulous technique, beveling incisions, breaking up a linear incision, and providing a tension-free closure.

Endoscopic Brow Lift

The minimally invasive endoscopic technique to forehead lifting was popularized by Isse[11] and is now the favored approach for many surgeons. It should be noted, however, that this approach involves a steep learning curve and specialized equipment. Multiple small skin incisions concealed posterior to the hairline are used to minimize risks including prominent scarring, alopecia, and anesthesia. The ideal patient for this approach has a normal to low hair line, relatively symmetric brow, mild to moderate brow ptosis, and minimal skin excess.[5] Although generally darker-skinned individuals and those with high hair lines or male pattern baldness were thought to be poor candidates for this procedure, with increased experience these patients may experience excellent outcomes from a minimally invasive surgery.[12] Varying number of incisions may be used to obtain adequate access and is based on surgeon preference, although typically five incisions are made in most patients placed approximately 0.5 to 1 cm posterior to the hairline.[3,13] Two vertical incisions are placed in the lateral temporal region, two obliquely oriented incisions in the lateral frontal region, and one horizontal incision in the midline. This allows for excellent access to all areas of concerns and generation of one large optical cavity for improved visualization. A subperiosteal dissection may then be performed in the midline, continuing superficial to the deep temporal fascia. This requires release of the conjoined tendon. A full release of the arcus marginalis is possible and

the corrugator and procerus muscles may be safely sectioned by this approach. The supraorbital and supratrochlear neurovascular bundles, sentinel vein, and temporal branch of the facial nerve may be identified and protected. Many different brow fixation or stabilization techniques have been used and are beyond the scope of this article.

COMPLICATIONS IN BROW LIFT

Overall, complication rates are typically low for any brow lift approach. One review of 393 patients undergoing primary or secondary endoscopic brow lift, 50% of whom had concomitant blepharoplasty, noted alopecia in one occurrence, transient scalp numbness in most patients, 2% with prolonged dysesthesia, and seven patients (almost 2%) with a temporary temporal nerve paresis.[14] A small forehead hematoma requiring in-office drainage occurred in 3.5% of patients. Seven percent of their patients experienced lagophthalmos, 8% with upper eyelid asymmetry, and 3% with brow malposition.

Bleeding

Bleeding complications may occur with any approach. These may be arterial, venous, or from skin edges. Preoperative patient education and avoidance of thinning agents is critical. Adequate injection with a hemostatic agent, obtaining intraoperative hemostasis, and avoidance of injury to the superficial temporal or zygomaticotemporal arteries, supraorbital or supratrochlear vascular bundles, and sentinel vein improves outcomes. If an injury to these structures is noted, it should be controlled before suspension and closure. Slow postoperative bleeding may be controlled with pressure alone, although hematomas necessitate evacuation and control of bleeding.

Nerve Injury

Anesthesia of the forehead should be discussed during the informed consent process. Although peri-incisional ansesthesia is expected, this should be temporary. The supratrochlear and supraorbital neurovascular bundles should be identified and preserved to minimize additional forehead hypoesthesia medially up to the vertex. Direct injury is uncommon; however, traction neuropraxia may occur secondary to suspension.[3] Temporally, dissection in a plane superficial to the superficial layer of the deep temporal fascia minimizes injury to the zygomaticotemporal and auriculotemporal branches of the second division of the trigeminal nerve and avoids temporal and lateral frontal parasthesias.[2]

Additionally, in the temporal region, great care must be taken to avoid injury to the temporal branch of the facial nerve because this results in paralysis and asymmetry of the forehead. Dissection in the plane superficial to the superficial layer of the deep temporal fascia and identification and preservation of the sentinel vein is important to protect this motor nerve.

Scarring and Alopecia

Prominent scarring and alopecia often discussed with open approaches typically results from poor incision and closure technique. This complication may be minimized in open approaches by making an irregular incision with an extreme bevel 4 to 5 mm posterior to the hairline in an area of consistent follicular density to avoid dermal appendages and allow for postoperative hair follicle growth through and around the forming scar.[15]

Brow Asymmetry and Over/Under Elevation

Postoperative brow asymmetries may cause poor patient satisfaction. Pre-existing asymmetries should be noted, photographically documented, and discussed with patients. Postoperative asymmetry may be caused by unrecognized preoperative asymmetries or blepharoptosis with failure.[13] Iatrogenic causes include asymmetric muscle resection or suspension. Proper patient selection, full bilateral release of the conjoined tendon and arcus marginalis, and symmetric suspension or skin excisions should be used to minimize this risk.

Overelevation or underelevation of the brow may occur with any approach to forehead rejuvenation.[13] Overresection of skin in any variation of the coronal lift or excessive suspension with any technique may result in overelevation of brow with possible lagophthalmos. This may be temporary and resolve with time or uncommonly may be permanent and difficult to address. This risk is increased when concomitant upper blepharoplasty is performed. The forehead lift should always precede eyelid surgery and overexcision of eyelid skin should be avoided. Lagophthalmos may cause symptoms of dryness or irritation and should be treated with lubricating eye drops and ointments. Limiting postoperative lagophthalmos to less than 2 mm is advised to decrease the risk of dry eye syndrome.[9] With proper careful technique, this complication may be avoided. In one series of 600 patients undergoing concomitant coronal brow lift and blepharoplasty, no occurrences of globe exposure, vision loss, or dry eye syndrome occurred and only two occurrences of brow asymmetry were noted.[7] Additionally, Dayan and colleagues[16] retrospectively compared the outcomes of patients who underwent either the endoscopic-assisted approach to the coronal or pretrichial forhead lift. They identified 140 patients of 400 who had at least 12 months of follow-up (121 coronal and 19 endoscopic). They noted no significant difference in brow elevation with either approach alone or in combination with blepharoplasty.

If excessive and caused by oversuspension, revision surgery with release of the suspension should be considered. Underelevation of the brow is likely secondary to inadequate release, suspension, or fixation. Unlike overelevation, this problem is more easily treated with revision brow lift and increasing the release, suspension, or skin resection. Overresection of the corrugator and procerus muscles may cause excessive medial brow elevation and a persistent "surprised" appearance and should be recognized and avoided. A more conservative approach to the glabellar musculature may be combined with postoperative adjunctive neuromodulation if needed.

SUMMARY

Forehead rejuvenation has had many advances from the traditional coronal lift to trichophytic and pretrichophytic modification, and in the past two decades has incorporated endoscopic approach as a popular means to provide long-lasting results with low complications. Overall, complications can be minimized by a thorough preoperative history and physical examination combined with meticulous technique, conservative suspension, and a tension-free wound closure.

REFERENCES

1. O'Brien JX, Ashton MW, Rozen WM, et al. New perspectives on the surgical anatomy and nomenclature of the temporal region: literature review and dissection study. Plast Reconstr Surg 2013;131(3): 510–22.
2. Knize DM. Anatomic concepts for brow lift procedures. Plast Reconstr Surg 2009;124(6):2118–26.
3. Terella AM, Wang TD. Technical considerations in endoscopic brow lift. Clin Plast Surg 2013;40(1): 105–15.
4. Sabini P, Wyne I, Quatela VC. Anatomical guides to precisely localize the frontal branch of the facial nerve. Arch Facial Plast Surg 2003;5:150–2.
5. Angelos PC, Stallworth CL, Wang TD. Forehead lifting: state of the art. Facial Plast Surg 2011;27(1): 050–7.

6. Pflugfelder SC, Solomon A, Stern ME. The diagnosis and management of dry eye: a twenty-five-year review. Cornea 2000;19(5):644–9.

7. Friedland JA, Jacobsen WM, TerKonda S. Safety and efficacy of combined upper blepharoplasties and open coronal browlift: a consecutive series of 600 patients. Aesthetic Plast Surg 1996;20(6):453–62.

8. Fagien S. Evaluation of the cosmetic oculoplastic surgery patient. In: Putterman's Cosmetic Oculoplastic Surgery. Ch 3. 4th edition. Philadelphia: Elsevier Saunders; 2007. p. 21–30.

9. Terella AM, Wang TD, Kim MM. Complications in periorbital surgery. Facial Plast Surg 2013;29(1):64–70.

10. Friedman O, Zaldivar RA, Wang TD. Blepharoplasty. In: Cummings otolaryngology: head & neck surgery. Ch 30. 5th edition. Philadelphia: Mosby/Elsevier; 2010. p. 439–51.

11. Isse NG. Endoscopic facial rejuvenation: endoforehead, the functional lift: case reports. Aesthetic Plast Surg 1994;18(1):21–9.

12. Shipchandler TZ, Sultan B, Byrne PJ. Endoscopic forehead lift in patients with male pattern baldness. Am J Otolaryngol 2012;33(5):519–22.

13. Guyuron B. Endoscopic forehead rejuvenation: I. Limitations, flaws, and rewards. Plast Reconstr Surg 2006;117(4):1121–33.

14. De Cordier BC, de la Torre JI, Al-Hakeem MS, et al. Endoscopic forehead lift: review of technique, cases, and complications. Plast Reconstr Surg 2002;110(6):1558–68.

15. Owsley TG. Subcutaneous trichophytic forehead browlift: the case for an "open" approach. J Oral Maxillofac Surg 2006;64(7):1133–6.

16. Dayan SH, Perkins SW, Vartanian AJ, et al. The forehead lift: endoscopic versus coronal approaches. Aesthetic Plast Surg 2001;25(1):35–9.

Recognizing and Managing Complications in Blepharoplasty

Katherine M. Whipple, MD, Bobby S. Korn, MD, PhD,
Don O. Kikkawa, MD*

KEYWORDS

- Cosmetic blepharoplasty • Upper eyelid blepharoplasty • Lower eyelid blepharoplasty
- Complications • Eyelid retraction • Dry eye • Exposure keratopathy

KEY POINTS

- Always err on the conservative side, as it is far easier to remove more tissue than to replace deficient tissue.
- Be patient during the healing process; time heals many imperfections and avoid early interventions.
- Proper preoperative counseling of patients is essential to maximize patient satisfaction with surgery.
- Preoperative and prior patient photographs are necessary to review before surgery and also help to document improvement.
- Upper eyelid markings are crucial to achieving optimal results and many complications can be avoided with proper markings.

INTRODUCTION

The earliest attempts at removing excess skin, puffiness, and wrinkling of the eyelid skin was during the tenth and eleventh centuries by Arabic surgeons.[1] Today, blepharoplasty has become the second most common cosmetic procedure performed in the United States.[2] It is one of the least invasive cosmetic surgeries available and, when performed correctly, is very safe and yields excellent results. It is one of the most effective ways to rejuvenate the periocular area. However, devastating complications, ranging from permanent vision loss to cosmetic deformity can occur following blepharoplasty. Most complications result from unrecognized changes in anatomy, errors in measurements, or overzealous removal of tissue (**Table 1**). This article outlines the most common blepharoplasty complications that occur, and offers preventive measures to avoid such complications.

INADVERTENT ERRORS IN ASSESSMENT

Residual Skin Excess

A conservative approach to blepharoplasty is essential, as the consequences of overaggressive tissue removal are more difficult to correct than the consequences of residual skin excess. Patients should be counseled preoperatively that approximately 5% to 10% of patients will need additional residual skin removed following blepharoplasty and that removing more skin later does not limit the final cosmetic result. Residual dermatochalasis usually results from an underestimation of

Supported generously by Steve and Kathleen Flynn and the Bell Charitable Foundation.
Division of Oculofacial Plastic and Reconstructive Surgery, University of California at San Diego, 9415 Campus Point Drive, La Jolla, CA 92093, USA
* Corresponding author.
E-mail address: dkikkawa@ucsd.edu

Facial Plast Surg Clin N Am 21 (2013) 625–637
http://dx.doi.org/10.1016/j.fsc.2013.08.002
1064-7406/13/$ – see front matter © 2013 Elsevier Inc. All rights reserved.

facialplastic.theclinics.com

Table 1
Causes, avoidance and correction of blepharoplasty complications

Complication	Causes	Avoidance	Correction
Residual upper lid skin	Underestimation of dermatochalasis	Learn and use proper pinch technique	Revision with skin excision
Eyelid ptosis	Unrecognized preoperatively, trauma to levator aponeurosis during blepharoplasty	Measure MRD preoperatively	Surgical correction of ptosis
Superior sulcus deformity	Overaggressive removal of fat during blepharoplasty	Evaluate superior sulcus preoperatively; judicious fat excision, medial only	Augment superior sulcus with fillers (autologous, hyaluronic acid)
Eyelid crease asymmetry	Uneven marking of eyelid crease	Measure eyelid crease with caliper at various points across lid	Crease revision with fixation to levator aponeurosis
Eyelid retraction/ectropion	Overly aggressive skin removal, scarring of the middle lamella	Conservative skin excision; minimize cautery	Middle lamellar release with posterior lamellar grafting
Canthal webbing	Extending incision too close to lid margin medially or laterally	Proper marking preoperatively	Z-plasty, canthoplasty, skin grafting
Brow ptosis	Unrecognized preoperatively; overaggressive skin removal from upper eyelid accentuates brow ptosis	Evaluate eyebrow position with patient in the relaxed state preoperatively	Correct eyebrow ptosis
Lagophthalmos	Overly aggressive skin removal from upper or lower eyelids	Conservative removal of skin	Full-thickness skin grafting; midface lifting, posterior/middle lamellar grafting
Globe perforation	Misdirection of needle during injection of local anesthetic	Never direct needle at globe	Emergent referral to ophthalmologist for complete eye examination
Hemorrhage (preseptal, retrobulbar)	Excessive venous or arterial hemorrhage	Stop anticoagulation; ensure surgical field is dry; avoid valsalva	Emergent canthotomy/cantholysis (retrobulbar); conservative measures (preseptal hematoma)
Infection (preseptal, orbital)	Bacterial, fungal	Prep with betadine; instruct patient to keep area clean and dry; antibiotic ointment	Preseptal: Trial of broad-spectrum oral antibiotics Orbital: Admit to hospital for intravenous antibiotics; ophthalmology consult
Diplopia	Traumatic injury to extraocular muscles; injection of local anesthetic into extraocular muscles; suture incorporation of muscle	Avoid deep injection	Referral to strabismus specialist
Lacrimal gland injury	Inadvertent resection of the lacrimal gland	Recognize appearance of lacrimal gland prolapse	Supportive measures with artificial tears, ointments

(continued on next page)

Table 1
(continued)

Complication	Causes	Avoidance	Correction
Horizontal eyelid phimosis	Lateral canthal dehiscence	Ensure lower crux of canthus is reapproximated to superior crux	Canthus-sparing canthopexy/canthoplasty
Corneal abrasion	Exposed cornea during surgery; accidental trauma during surgery	Corneal protectors with ointment	Referral to ophthalmologist
Fire	Spontaneous combustion of flammable material, spark, and oxygen	Avoid use of cautery, moisten field during cautery use, turn off supplemental oxygen	Supportive measures
Wound dehiscence	Poorly tied sutures, patient noncompliance (rubbing, exertion)	Proper suture technique	Debride wound and resuture
Suture granuloma	Foreign body reaction to suture	Use smallest sutures possible	Observation, trial of steroid cream, excision
The dissatisfied patient	Unrealistic expectations, unexpected bruising or postoperative healing, personality difference	Full disclosure of risks of surgery, realistic expectations of surgery	Reassurance, empathy frequent office visits

how much dermatochalasis is present and is noted most commonly on the lateral eyelid.

In any patient desiring further removal of eyelid skin, evaluation for eyebrow ptosis should be performed. If concurrent eyebrow ptosis is present, removal of more skin will only exaggerate the eyebrow ptosis. For these patients, the eyebrow ptosis should be addressed before revising the blepharoplasty. If eyebrow ptosis is not present, the surgeon must ensure adequate skin remains for the eyelid to properly close after revision. Historically, this has been 20 mm measured in the center of the eyelid, from the lash line to the base of the brow. If the patient has cosmetically altered the brows with tattoos, the natural brow height should be used.

Patients may request more skin to be removed when there is questionable residual skin present. Explanation of the importance of proper lid function and avoidance of lagophthalmos informs the patient of additional risk and usually dissuades the patient from seeking further revision. Revision should be considered only after healing is complete, usually 3 to 6 months after the initial surgery.

Eyelid Ptosis

If unrecognized, uncorrected eyelid ptosis limits the cosmetic result of a blepharoplasty. Ptosis is defined medically as a margin-to-reflex distance-1

of 2.5 mm or less. However, many patients recognize even more subtle differences between the eyelid heights, and even as little as 0.5 mm will be intolerable to some patients. Therefore, the margin-to-reflex distance must be measured preoperatively with the patient in the relaxed state to document asymmetry. Preoperative discussion with the patient regarding preexisting ptosis is essential to avoid postoperative disappointment.

In the early postoperative period, eyelid ptosis following blepharoplasty is not uncommon. It can be the result of postoperative edema and should not be worrisome; however, if ptosis persists after resolution of postoperative edema, it is possible the levator muscle/aponeurosis was traumatized or disinserted during blepharoplasty (**Fig. 1**). If the levator function is decreased following surgery, damage to the muscle should be expected and likely the patient will require levator advancement to correct the ptosis. Sound knowledge of the eyelid anatomy is essential to avoid inadvertent damage to surrounding structures. The levator muscle is located directly beneath the preaponeurotic fat pad; therefore, dissection beyond the fat pads should be limited to avoid levator injury (**Fig. 2**).

Superior Sulcus Contour Deformity/Hollowing

Trends in upper and lower blepharoplasty rejuvenation techniques have shifted from fat resection

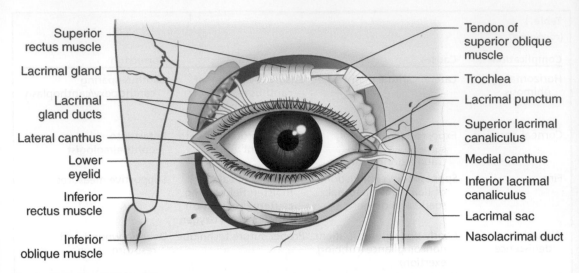

Fig. 1. Anatomy of the orbit.

Superior rectus muscle

Lacrimal gland

Lacrimal gland ducts

Lateral canthus

Lower eyelid

Inferior rectus muscle

Inferior oblique muscle

Tendon of superior oblique muscle

Trochlea

Lacrimal punctum

Superior lacrimal canaliculus

Medial canthus

Inferior lacrimal canaliculus

Lacrimal sac

Nasolacrimal duct

to fat conservation.[3,4] A youthful upper eyelid is full, especially in the lateral aspect.[5] With time, the central fat pad atrophies, while the medial fat pad become more prominent; this can cause a tear drop–shaped deformity in an otherwise hollowed eyelid (**Fig. 3**).[6] Overaggressive resection of fat during upper eyelid blepharoplasty can result in a hollowed superior sulcus that is particularly aging. The volume of the upper eyelid is in part

made up of the medial and central fat pads, as well as the eyebrow fat pad. The composition of these fat pads is different. The medial fat pad is lighter in color due to variations in carotenoid composition and possibly from enrichment of orbital stem cells.[7,8] Targeted removal or repositioning of the medial upper eyelid fat may be necessary if a patient has a tear drop nasal fat accumulation.[9–11] Preoperative examination

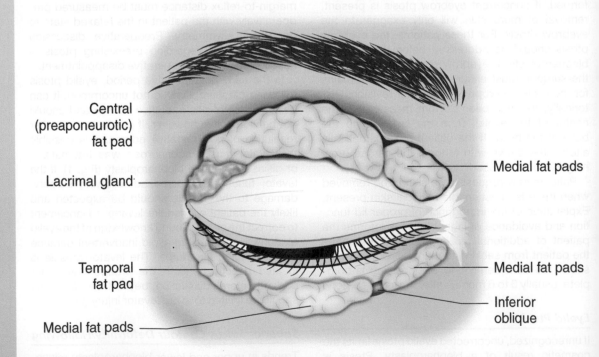

Central (preaponeurotic) fat pad

Lacrimal gland

Temporal fat pad

Medial fat pads

Medial fat pads

Medial fat pads

Inferior oblique

Fig. 2. Fat pads of the upper and lower eyelid.

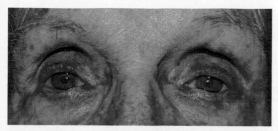

Fig. 3. Natural hollowing of the upper eyelids in an 89-year-old Caucasian woman. No eyelid surgery has been performed.

should include observation of the medial and lateral eyelid contour to evaluate the prominence of the medial and central fat pads.

Asymmetric Eyelid Crease

Although there are studies both for and against symmetry equaling beauty in a face, almost all faces have some asymmetry.[12] Patients seeking cosmetic or functional blepharoplasty, however, expect relative symmetry postoperatively. After blepharoplasty, some patients will notice asymmetry between their eyes that was present preoperatively, but never recognized. For this reason, it is essential to have high-quality preoperative photographs documenting asymmetry.

However, errors in preoperative assessment and markings, in some cases, may lead to avoidable asymmetry postoperatively (Fig. 4). Complete preoperative examination of eyelids for ptosis, globe prominence, and thyroid eye disease is necessary to avoid suboptimal results.

Marking of the skin is the most critical portion of the upper eyelid blepharoplasty surgery. Although there are standard guidelines, the markings are for the most part artistic and decided on by the surgeon. Some variations in markings exist that will yield slight differences in results, but in general the better outcome is in the eye of the beholder (Fig. 5). Usually, respecting the patient's natural eyelid crease is desired, unless the patient wishes an altered lid crease. If no obvious crease is visible or if the crease is heightened due to levator dehiscence, marking the eyelid crease 7 to 8 mm above the lash line in Caucasian men and 8 to 10 mm

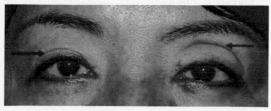

Fig. 4. Asymmetric eyelid creases (black arrows) following blepharoplasty.

above the lash line in Caucasian women yields are good guidelines. Guidelines in Asian men are a crease set between 5 to 6 mm and Asian women at 6 to 7 mm.

The crease extends in a fairly mild arc from lateral to medial canthus. Beyond the puncta, the marking should angle superiorly to avoid medial canthal webbing postoperatively. Laterally, beyond the lateral canthus, the marking should also angle superiorly to address any hooding. Then, 2 nontoothed forceps should be used to pinch the excess skin while avoiding lagophthalmos. This should be performed centrally, medially, and laterally to mark the redundant skin. These points should then be connected in a smooth arc. The patient is then asked to open his or her eyelids and the upper and lower markings should blend together (see Fig. 5C).

Initially, asymmetry between the eyelids is common and the patient can be reassured. However, once the healing is complete, if significant asymmetry exists, revision may be considered. In general, it is easier to raise a crease rather than lowering one. A higher crease may be created by making a new incision above the previous mark and fixating the orbicularis at the new height to the levator aponeurosis. Lowering the crease is more difficult, and requires making a lower incision at the new lower level with advancement of the preaponeurotic fat or placing free fat pearls to prevent readhesion at the higher level. Although good results can be obtained, these results are often not as desirable as appropriate initial marking.

Eyelid Retraction/Ectropion

One of the most troublesome complications following lower eyelid blepharoplasty is eyelid retraction and cicatricial ectropion, as they are not only cosmetically deforming, but can cause agonizing symptoms of foreign body sensation and decreased vision (Fig. 6A). Eyelid retraction often results from scarring of the middle lamella during lower eyelid blepharoplasty. Eyelid ectropion is typically caused by aggressive removal of skin during lower eyelid blepharoplasty and unrecognized lower eyelid laxity. To avoid this, judicious skin removal should be performed during lower eyelid blepharoplasty only if significant redundancy of the skin exists. In general, at most only a few millimeters of skin should be removed. Many patients only require lower eyelid fat recontouring rather than skin excision. It is important to explain to patients preoperatively that lower eyelid blepharoplasty addresses the contour of the lower eyelid rather than removal of skin. The crepelike quality and deep rhytids of the skin will

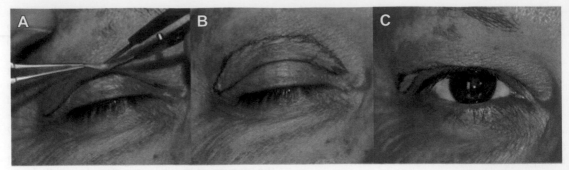

Fig. 5. Eyelid blepharoplasty markings. (A) The lower mark usually courses along the patient's natural eyelid crease and nontoothed forceps are used to grasp the redundant skin with the lower forceps grasping at the inferior mark. (B) The completed mark for upper eyelid blepharoplasty. (C) As a guideline, usually the potential skin to be removed should "disappear" when patients open their eyes.

not change with blepharoplasty. Often a skin treatment, such as a chemical peel or laser resurfacing, is needed to address this.

Correction of eyelid retraction can be performed with autologous tissue, such as hard palate, dermis fat, or acellular dermis, to build up the posterior with complete release of the middle lamella (see **Fig. 6**B).[13–16] Skin grafting is considered the last option and will likely be necessary only in severe cases. Although reconstructive efforts result in restored lid position, often the function and cosmetic result is not as ideal as if the retraction and ectropion did not occur.

Canthal Webbing

An unsightly complication following blepharoplasty is webbing of the tissue at the medial or lateral canthus. Medially, this often results from the incision nearing the lid margin too closely or if the incision is extended to far medially or

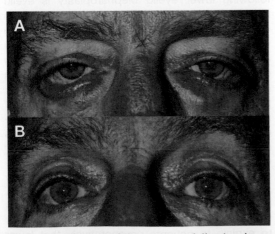

Fig. 6. (A) Severe eyelid retraction following lower eyelid blepharoplasty. (B) Postoperative photo demonstrating correction of the lower eyelid retraction with Enduragen implant to both lower eyelids.

inappropriately angled inferiorly. Laterally, this results when the upper and lower incisions join to create an inferior angle or if too much skin is removed. This is more likely to occur in Asian patients, or any patient with a lower-set eyelid crease and patients with brow ptosis. Proper marking is essential to avoid this complication.

Brow Ptosis

Accurate preoperative assessment of the facial and eyelid anatomy is essential to achieving a sound cosmetic result. Identification of the eyebrow ptosis preoperatively is essential. Regardless of the amount of skin to be removed during blepharoplasty, at least 20 mm of skin should remain on the upper eyelid to allow for proper eyelid closure following surgery. If brow ptosis is unrecognized and the amount of remaining skin is not measured, excessive skin can be removed, leading to lagophthalmos and further exaggeration of the eyebrow ptosis (**Fig. 7**). This is a difficult problem to fix and may require skin grafting to ameliorate the problem. In cosmetic patients, this may not be an acceptable option, so supportive measures with aggressive lubrication should be initiated.

Lagophthalmos

Lagophthalmos, or the inability to close the eyelids following surgery, has various causes and usually is transient. Preoperatively, patients should be asked about previous eyelid and facial procedures. In particular, patients should be asked about previous eye surgery, such as laser in situ keratomileusis (LASIK), as these patients are more likely to develop symptoms from lagophthalmos following surgery.[17] Early postoperative lagophthalmos is usually due to edema, decreased patient effort because of pain, or temporary orbicularis dysfunction and usually resolves with

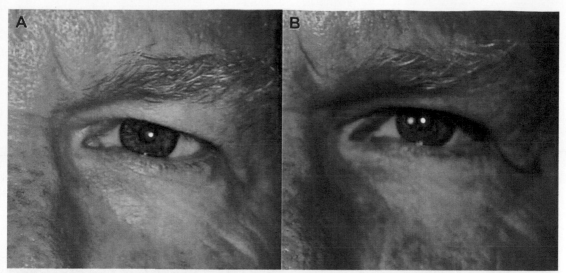

Fig. 7. (*A*) Preoperative photo of patient complaining of his eyelids blocking vision. (*B*) Postoperative photo following blepharoplasty only. The result was limited, as his brow ptosis was not corrected at the time of surgery.

time. Artificial tears and ointment may be necessary to ensure the cornea remains moisturized during this time. Persistent lagophthalmos extending beyond the postoperative period may require intervention. Patients may be able to tolerate mild lagophthalmos if they have an intact Bell phenomenon; however, more than 2 mm usually causes symptoms of tearing, foreign body sensation, conjunctival injection, corneal decompensation, and vision loss (**Fig. 8**).

Causes of lagophthalmos include excessive removal of skin from the upper eyelid, orbicularis paresis due to facial nerve injury, excessive orbicularis resection, and eyelid retraction. Accurate preoperative assessment of eyelid and facial relationships and conservative markings is key to avoiding lagophthalmos. At least 20 mm of skin should remain, when measured from brow to lid margin in the center of the eyelid, after the excess skin is excised, in order for the lid to close properly (**Fig. 9**).

The cosmetic patient who wants every last bit of redundant skin removed should be counseled that this is not possible nor desired. Proper explanation

of the importance of eyelid function and reassurance that the primary goal of surgery is to improve appearance while respecting the role of the eyelids is often adequate to manage expectations. Also, informing patients that a touch up is possible to remove residual skin if necessary reassures them.

SURGICAL COMPLICATIONS
Inadvertent Globe Perforation

Use of local anesthetic is essential for patients during blepharoplasty, whether performed under intravenous sedation or general anesthesia. Our preference is to use a mixture of 0.375% marcaine mixed with 1% lidocaine with 1:200,000 epinephrine to anesthetize the eyelid and achieve hemostasis. Inadvertent perforation of the globe with the needle with subsequent injection of anesthetic is a devastating and avoidable complication.[18,19] On injection, the needle tip should always be directed away from the globe. Once in the subcutaneous space, the anesthetic should be injected slowly to create a fluid wave that separates the tissues, creating more room for the needle tip to be advanced. Traction can also be placed on the upper eyelid and brow to elevate the upper lid from the globe to give addition space.

Hemorrhage

Regardless of the technique used, a small amount of hemorrhage is expected during surgery, with resultant ecchymosis. Patients should be informed preoperatively of this to manage postoperative concerns. A thorough preoperative history should be taken, including anticoagulation use and herbal

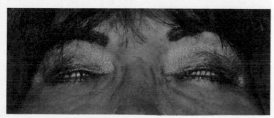

Fig. 8. Patient with lagophthalmos following overaggressive resection of eyelid skin.

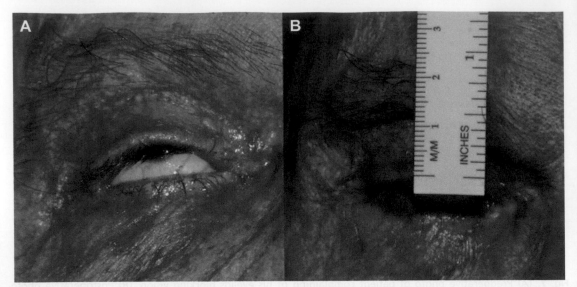

Fig. 9. (*A*) Postoperative image of a patient following blepharoplasty with lagophthalmos due to overaggressive resection of skin. (*B*) Only 12 mm of skin remains from his lash line to inferior brow.

supplements. To minimize bleeding during surgery, these medications should be discontinued if possible.[20,21] Some patients elect to take the herbal supplement, *Arnica montana*, in hopes to improve postoperative bruising; however, most evidence has been anecdotal.[22] One randomized trial of patients using *A montana* following face-lifts did show statistically significant improvement in postoperative ecchymosis.[23] However, in the only randomized, placebo-controlled study available evaluating the effectiveness of *A montana* following blepharoplasty, no statistically significant improvement was found.[24]

Preseptal Hematoma

Postoperatively, the residual or active hemorrhage may spread diffusely across the lid in the preseptal space or form a focal hematoma. This may result in an unsightly, swollen, sometime tense lid (**Fig. 10**). In these cases, it is essential to evaluate for a retrobulbar hematoma (discussed later in this article). In a preseptal hematoma, the vision is usually not compromised and pain is minimal. If the hematoma is deemed to be located only in the preseptal space, direct pressure and cold compresses should be applied. Preseptal hematomas are best managed with conservative measures, such as keeping the head elevated, applying ice, rest, and close observation. Attempts to evacuate or drain the hematoma is typically not necessary and may cause recurrent bleeding. The tension created in the preseptal space by the hematoma may tamponade the leaking vessel. Therefore, removal of the hematoma may cause recurrent

accumulation. Preseptal hematoma is often very concerning to the patient due to delayed recovering and its appearance; however, they are rarely a threat to vision and to the final esthetic outcome. It is essential to counsel patients of this before surgery and if it does occur, reassure patients that the hematoma will resolve and the result will likely not be compromised.

Retrobulbar Hematoma

A retrobulbar hemorrhage is one of the most feared consequences of blepharoplasty (**Fig. 11**).

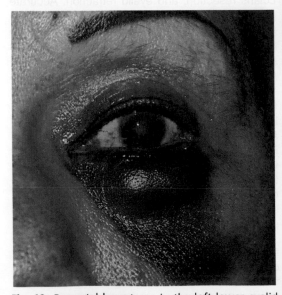

Fig. 10. Preseptal hematoma in the left lower eyelid following lower eyelid blepharoplasty.

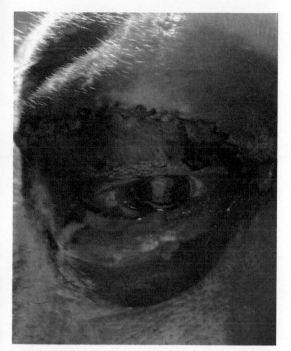

Fig. 11. Retrobulbar hematoma occurring 12 hours after blepharoplasty.

Fortunately, this complication is rare, with an incidence of 0.055%. Permanent vision loss following blepharoplasty is even more rare, with an incidence of 0.045%.[25] Although most occur within 24 hours days after surgery, retrobulbar hemorrhages leading to permanent vision loss have been reported up to 9 days postoperatively.[26] During blepharoplasty, the septum is often opened to remove or reposition the preaponeurotic fat pad. This creates a communication between the anterior and posterior orbit and a track for blood to travel into the orbit. Usually, retrobulbar hematoma is caused by arterial bleeding, either superficial or deep. The orbital volume is 30 mL, with little room for tissue expansion. Therefore, blood accumulation can lead to a compartment syndrome, with severe pain, proptosis, limitation of extraocular movements, increased intraocular pressure, and an afferent pupillary defect if the optic nerve is compressed. Vision loss can occur, as the vascular supply to the retina is compromised from increased pressure. It represents a true ophthalmic emergency. If the orbital compartment syndrome if not addressed, vision loss can be permanent.

If signs of retrobulbar hemorrhage are present following surgery, an emergent lateral canthotomy/cantholysis should be performed. Initially, the diagnosis of a retrobulbar hemorrhage is a clinical one, and the decision to perform canthotomy/cantholysis should not be delayed for radiographic studies to confirm findings. Complete release of the inferior crus should be performed first. The upper crus can be lysed as well, if needed. Once the canthotomy/cantholysis has been performed, the surgical wound should be explored for the offending vessel and cautery applied.

Preseptal/Orbital Cellulitis

The vascular supply to the eyelid is robust and fortunately, postoperative infections are rare. The most common pathogens are *Staphylococcus* and *Streptococcus* species.[27] However, more unusual pathogens may invade the eyelids, including atypical mycobacteria. Necrotizing fasciitis has also been reported.[28,29] Additionally, methicillin-resistant *Staphylococcus aureus* has been an increasing source of postoperative infections following any surgery, including blepharoplasty.[30] If untreated, infections can spread rapidly and cause permanent vision loss, so early diagnosis and treatment are essential. Certain groups of patients, such as immunosuppressed patients, are at increased risk of developing infections postoperatively.

If localized to the preseptal space, infection can be managed empirically as an outpatient with broad-spectrum antibiotics and close follow-up (**Fig. 12**). Presenting symptoms usually include erythema around the incision, heat, swelling, and discharge. Vision is usually unaffected, extraocular movements are normal, the pupils react normally, there is no chemosis, and proptosis is not present. If any of these findings are present, orbital cellulitis should be suspected and the patient should be

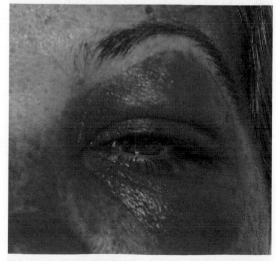

Fig. 12. Preseptal cellulitis of the left upper eyelid demonstrating erythema and edema of skin. The edges of the cellulitis were marked with a pen to ensure the infection was improving daily.

treated more aggressively. This includes hospital admission for intravenous antibiotics, a complete examination by an ophthalmologist, and radiographic imaging to evaluate for the presence of an orbital abscess and extent of infection.[27] If an orbital abscess is present and vision is compromised, the abscess should be drained surgically as soon as possible. If the vision is stable, intravenous antibiotics can be started and the patient monitored closely for improvement. In most cases, the patient requires 24 to 48 hours of antibiotics before clinical improvement will be seen. If there is no improvement or any evidence of deterioration, surgical drainage should be undertaken.

Atypical mycobacterial infections should be suspected when delayed wound infections present or multiple erythematous lesions are present. Cultures should be taken with appropriate culture media and an infectious disease consult may be required. Cultures can take weeks to be positive and systemic macrolides are typically necessary to eradicate the infection (**Fig. 13**).

Diplopia

If a patient complains of double vision following upper and/or lower eyelid blepharoplasty, it is important to determine whether the diplopia is monocular or binocular. Monocular diplopia results from previous refractive error tear film disruption, corneal injury, or ointment. Binocular diplopia immediately following surgery may be due to infiltration of extraocular muscles with local anesthetic.[31,32] This can rarely lead to toxicity of the

affected muscle, causing hypertrophy and fibrosis of the muscle, ultimately leading to diplopia in the opposite direction than it initially presented. Reversal of the diplopia postoperatively is suggestive of anesthetic infiltration of an extraocular muscle.[33] This is often seen with lower eyelid anesthesia as inferior rectus muscle function may be transiently diminished. In the early postoperative period, binocular diplopia may also be due to normal postoperative edema and will resolve as the edema improves. However, if diplopia persists in the postoperative period, referral to an ophthalmologist is warranted for a complete evaluation. The trochlea, or pulley of the superior oblique, is located just behind the orbital rim and can become damaged or scarred during aggressive nasal fat pad removal, leading to an iatrogenic Brown syndrome.[34] In the lower eyelid, the inferior oblique travels between the medial and central eyelid and can easily be transected or cauterized during fat recontouring.[35] In addition, fat redraping sutures may inadvertently incorporate the muscle or its fascial sheath. Strabismus surgery may be required to realign the eyes if the ocular deviation persists.

Lacrimal Gland Injury

The upper eyelid contains 2 fat pads: the medial and the preaponeurotic fat pads. The lacrimal gland rests in the lacrimal gland fossa, located just posterior to superolateral orbital rim and lateral to the preaponeurotic fat pad (**Fig. 14**). It functions as part of the accessory lacrimal system. The incidence of lacrimal gland prolapse had traditionally been described as approximately 10% to 15% of patients.[36] However, more recent reports indicate the incidence may be as high as 60%.[37]

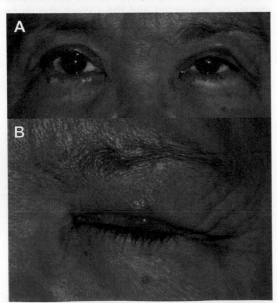

Fig. 13. (A) Left upper eyelid atypical mycobacterial infection following blepharoplasty. (B) Enlarged view of the infected area.

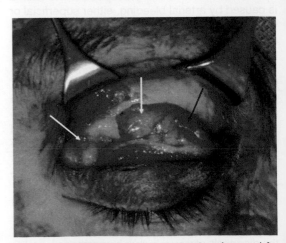

Fig. 14. Left upper eyelid demonstrating the nasal fat pat (*white arrow*), the central or preaponeurotic fat pad (*yellow arrow*), and lacrimal gland (*black arrow*).

With relaxation of the orbital tissues, the lacrimal gland may prolapse forward, creating a bulge in the superolateral eyelid contour. Thorough understanding of the eyelid anatomy is key, and it is essential to not mistake a prolapsed lacrimal gland as fat. Removal or damage to the lacrimal gland can lead to dacryops formation, dry eye, foreign body sensation, corneal decompensation, and vision loss. If a prolapsed lacrimal gland is identified preoperatively, it can easily be repositioned back into the lacrimal gland fossa.

Horizontal Eyelid Phimosis

Horizontal phimosis can occur following lower eyelid blepharoplasty due to horizontal contractile forces and also if the lateral canthus is disinserted from the orbital rim. It can lead to shortening of the horizontal fissure, giving patients a "small-eyed" look that is unacceptable, and may also cause tearing from poor lacrimal outflow (**Fig. 15**). It is generally accepted that the area of sclera visible laterally from the cornea should be larger than the area of sclera medial to the cornea. Horizontal laxity often needs to be addressed at the time of lower eyelid blepharoplasty. Some patients undergoing lower lid blepharoplasty require tightening of the lower eyelid, either in the form of canthopexy or canthoplasty. If present postoperatively, correction is possible through a canthus-sparing canthopexy.

Corneal Abrasion

A corneal abrasion results from disruption of the corneal epithelium. This should be suspected when a patient complains of severe eye pain and tearing immediately following surgery and more serious complications (eg, retrobulbar hematoma) have been ruled out. Corneal abrasions usually occur from exposure of the cornea during a surgery or inadvertent injury to the epithelium during surgery. Corneal injury can be avoided by careful placement of corneal protectors with ointment into both operated and nonoperated eyes at the beginning of the case.

Diagnosis is confirmed with fluorescein and a cobalt blue light. Once diagnosed, the treatment may include lubrication, patching, and a bandage contact lens. Although the corneal epithelium is very sensitive, it also heals very quickly. An ophthalmologist should see patients with corneal abrasions daily until the defect has completely resolved to prevent progression into a corneal ulcer.

Fire/Burned Skin/Lashes

There are approximately 100 intraoperative fires annually, with 15% resulting in serious injuries (**Fig. 16**).[38] Increasing use of electric cautery has been blamed with the increase in intraoperative fires since 1994; however, oxygen cannulas, and use of ethanol-based products and disposable drapes are contributing factors.[39] To decrease the risk of fire, the surgeon should ensure the nasal cannula is above the drape to avoid an oxygen trap. If possible, the oxygen should be turned off when cautery is being used. The lashes and brow cilia should be moistened before cautery use. Finally, removal of saponified fat should be performed throughout eyelid fat pad sculpting and repositioning to lessen the risk.

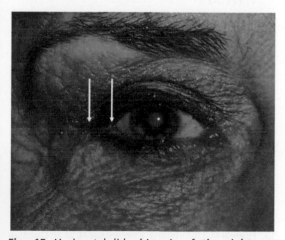

Fig. 15. Horizontal lid phimosis of the right eye following canthoplasty. The lateral canthus (*white arrow*) should rest closer to the orbital rim (*yellow arrow*). Note that the area of sclera lateral to the cornea is smaller than the area of the sclera medial to the cornea.

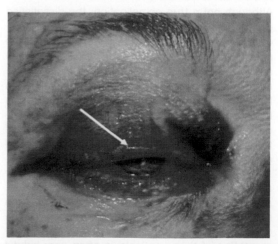

Fig. 16. Singed lashes (*yellow arrow*) of the right upper eyelid following intraoperative fire during lower eyelid blepharoplasty.

Wound Dehiscence

Many techniques exist on blepharoplasty closure, and the technique used is dependent on surgeon preference. Our preference of closure involves approximation of the orbicularis using 7-0 polygalactin suture and skin closure with 6-0 fast-absorbing gut suture. Nonabsorbable sutures work well also, yet patients are pleased not to need suture removal postoperatively. Absorbable sutures can create inflammation during wound healing, but we have not found this to be problematic. Should a dehiscence occur, the area should be deepithelialized and resutured. Proper counseling of patients to ensure they are not lifting anything heavy, exercising, or lowering their head below their waist will decrease the amount of dehiscences that occur. If the dehisced area is smaller than 1 cm, the wound may be observed and allowed to close via secondary intention. Conservative measures, such as continuing ointment until the area is fully healed, is all that is needed and once healed, usually the area is unrecognizable.

Suture Granuloma

Focal inflammation around any suture may occur following blepharoplasty. This is more common at the medial and canthus, where knots are placed. Although not painful, they can be very noticeable to patients. Most granulomas resolve with time. Topical steroids may be used to attempt to decrease inflammation. Alternatively, they can be excised in the office.

The Dissatisfied Patient

Although not a true complication, the dissatisfied patient following blepharoplasty can be a significant source of aggravation for the surgeon in the postoperative period. To avoid this, reasonable surgical expectations should be discussed. Numerous preoperative photographs should be taken from various angles at the initial consultation and in the preoperative suite. Asymmetry should be addressed preoperatively. Thorough discussion of the true postoperative course should be discussed and expectations should be set.

Patients often adapt very quickly to their new appearance and often forget where they started. Additionally, after surgery most patients become more aware of "flaws" as they are looking more closely at the surgical area. Preoperative documentation of these patients is often very helpful to the surgeon to show that the imperfections were present preoperatively.

SUMMARY

There is an artistic element to blepharoplasty surgery, and no matter how prepared and experienced a surgeon is, perfect results are not always achievable. True perfection is unobtainable, because patients and their facial expressions are dynamic. However, expert knowledge of eyelid and facial anatomy, combined with the knowledge of common pitfalls of blepharoplasty as outlined in this article, will yield reproducible, consistent results and keep the eye and periocular tissues protected.

REFERENCES

1. Swaddle JP, Cuthill IC. Asymmetry and human facial attractiveness: symmetry may not always be beautiful. Proc Biol Sci 1995;261(1360):111–6.
2. International Communications Research. 2011 AAFPRS Membership Study. January 2012:1–35.
3. Hamra ST. The role of orbital fat preservation in facial aesthetic surgery. A new concept. Clin Plast Surg 1996;23:17–28.
4. Lam S, Glasgold M, Glasgold R. Complementary fat graphing. Philadelphia: Lippincott Williams & Wilkins; 2007.
5. Fezza JP. The sigmoid upper eyelid blepharoplasty: redefining beauty. Ophthal Plast Reconstr Surg 2012;28:446–51.
6. Oh SR, Chokthaweesak W, Annunziata CC, et al. Analysis of eyelid fat pad changes with aging. Ophthal Plast Reconstr Surg 2011;27:348–51.
7. Sires BS, Saari JC, Garwin GG, et al. The color difference in orbital fat. Arch Ophthalmol 2001; 119:868–71.
8. Korn BS, Kikkawa DO, Hicok KC. Identification and characterization of adult stem cells from human orbital adipose tissue. Ophthal Plast Reconstr Surg 2009;25:27–32.
9. Massry GG. Nasal fat preservation in upper eyelid blepharoplasty. Ophthal Plast Reconstr Surg 2011; 27:352–5.
10. Lee JW, Baker SR. Esthetic enhancements in upper blepharoplasty. Clin Plast Surg 2013;40:139–46.
11. Oh SR, Chokthaweesak W, Annunziata CC, et al. Analysis of eyelid fat pad changes with aging. Ophthal Plast Reconstr Surg 2011;27(5):348–51.
12. Swaddle JP, Cuthill IC. Asymmetry and human facial attractiveness: symmetry may not always be beautiful. Proc Biol Sci 1995;261:111–6.
13. Borrelli M, Unterlauft J, Kleinsasser N, et al. Decellularized porcine derived membrane (Tarsys(R)) for correction of lower eyelid retraction. Orbit 2012;31: 187–9.
14. Oestreicher JH, Pang NK, Liao W. Treatment of lower eyelid retraction by retractor release and posterior

lamellar grafting: an analysis of 659 eyelids in 400 patients. Ophthal Plast Reconstr Surg 2008;24: 207–12.

15. Korn BS, Kikkawa DO, Cohen SR. Transcutaneous lower eyelid blepharoplasty with orbitomalar suspension: retrospective review of 212 consecutive cases. Plast Reconstr Surg 2010;125:315–23.

16. Korn BS, Kikkawa DO, Cohen SR, et al. Treatment of lower eyelid malposition with dermis fat grafting. Ophthalmology 2008;115:744–51.e2.

17. Korn BS, Kikkawa DO, Schanzlin DJ. Blepharoplasty in the post-laser in situ keratomileusis patient: preoperative considerations to avoid dry eye syndrome. Plast Reconstr Surg 2007;119:2232–9.

18. Schrader WF, Schargus M, Schneider E, et al. Risks and sequelae of scleral perforation during peribulbar or retrobulbar anesthesia. J Cataract Refract Surg 2010;36:885–9.

19. Ghosh S, Mukhopadhyay S, Mukhopadhyay S, et al. Inadvertent intracorneal injection of local anesthetic during lid surgery. Cornea 2010;29:701–2.

20. Heller J, Gabbay JS, Ghadjar K, et al. Top-10 list of herbal and supplemental medicines used by cosmetic patients: what the plastic surgeon needs to know. Plast Reconstr Surg 2006;117:436–45 [discussion: 446–7].

21. Spyropoulos AC, Douketis JD, Gerotziafas G, et al. Periprocedural antithrombotic and bridging therapy: recommendations for standardized reporting in patients with arterial indications for chronic oral anticoagulant therapy. J Thromb Haemost 2012;10:692–4.

22. Riley D. Arnica montana and homeopathic dosing guidelines. Plast Reconstr Surg 2003;112:693.

23. Seeley BM, Denton AB, Ahn MS, et al. Effect of homeopathic Arnica montana on bruising in face-lifts: results of a randomized, double-blind, placebo-controlled clinical trial. Arch Facial Plast Surg 2006;8:54–9.

24. Kotlus BS, Heringer DM, Dryden RM. Evaluation of homeopathic Arnica montana for ecchymosis after upper blepharoplasty: a placebo-controlled, randomized, double-blind study. Ophthal Plast Reconstr Surg 2010;26:395–7.

25. Hass AN, Penne RB, Stefanyszyn MA, et al. Incidence of postblepharoplasty orbital hemorrhage and associated visual loss. Ophthal Plast Reconstr Surg 2004;20:426–32.

26. Teng CC, Reddy S, Wong JJ, et al. Retrobulbar hemorrhage nine days after cosmetic blepharoplasty resulting in permanent visual loss. Ophthal Plast Reconstr Surg 2006;22:388–9.

27. Chaudhry IA, Shamsi FA, Elzaridi E, et al. Outcome of treated orbital cellulitis in a tertiary eye care center in the Middle East. Ophthalmology 2007;114:345–54.

28. Mauriello JA Jr. Atypical mycobacterial infection of the periocular region after periocular and facial surgery. Ophthal Plast Reconstr Surg 2003;19:182–8.

29. Suner IJ, Meldrum ML, Johnson TE, et al. Necrotizing fasciitis after cosmetic blepharoplasty. Am J Ophthalmol 1999;128:367–8.

30. Juthani V, Zoumalan CI, Lisman RD, et al. Successful management of methicillin-resistant Staphylococcus aureus orbital cellulitis after blepharoplasty. Plast Reconstr Surg 2010;126:305e–7e.

31. Guyton DL. Strabismus complications from local anesthetics. Semin Ophthalmol 2008;23:298–301.

32. Rainin EA, Carlson BM. Postoperative diplopia and ptosis. A clinical hypothesis based on the myotoxicity of local anesthetics. Arch Ophthalmol 1985;103: 1337–9.

33. Capo H, Guyton DL. Ipsilateral hypertropia after cataract surgery. Ophthalmology 1996;103:721–30.

34. Wilde C, Batterbury M, Durnian J. Acquired Brown's syndrome following cosmetic blepharoplasty. Eye (Lond) 2012;26:757–8.

35. Pirouzian A, Goldberg RA, Demer JL. Inferior rectus pulley hindrance: a mechanism of restrictive hypertropia following lower lid surgery. J AAPOS 2004;8: 338–44.

36. Smith B, Lisman RD. Dacryoadenopexy as a recognized factor in upper lid blepharoplasty. Plast Reconstr Surg 1983;71:629–32.

37. Massry GG. Prevalence of lacrimal gland prolapse in the functional blepharoplasty population. Ophthal Plast Reconstr Surg 2011;27:410–3.

38. Haith LR Jr, Santavasi W, Shapiro TK, et al. Burn center management of operating room fire injuries. J Burn Care Res 2012;33:649–53.

39. Rinder CS. Fire safety in the operating room. Curr Opin Anaesthesiol 2008;21:790–5.

Complications of Rhinoplasty

Joshua B. Surowitz, MD*, Sam P. Most, MD

KEYWORDS

- Rhinoplasty • Septorhinoplasty • Complications

KEY POINTS

- Meticulous history, physical examination, and standardized photographic documentation are central to preoperative evaluation and surgical planning for rhinoplasty.
- Photographic documentation is very useful to help illustrate preexisting preoperative asymmetries, and the surgeon must document these in the physical examination and discuss them with the patient.
- As with any surgery, any complications should be openly discussed with the patient.
- Appropriate preoperative counseling regarding all risks, benefits, and alternatives is critical.
- The surgeon must have a comprehensive understanding of nasal anatomy and effects of surgical maneuvers to help avoid complications.

OVERVIEW

Rhinoplasty Is a very common surgical procedure among facial and general plastic surgeons. It may be performed for functional and aesthetic reasons. It is a highly technically challenging procedure, because the surgeon must pay careful attention to both form and function. An aesthetically pleasing nose without the ability to breathe is a surgical failure. Some complications may occur intraoperatively, whereas others may occur postoperatively during wound healing and contracture. Therefore, some complications may not become evident until months to years after surgery.

ASYMMETRIES

Asymmetries of the bony pyramid can occur for multiple reasons, including discrepancies in osteotomies between sides, asymmetric dorsal reduction, and persistence of preoperative asymmetries. A greenstick fracture, with failure to fully

osteotomize, may result in either failure to fully mobilize the nasal bone or the nasal bone lateralizing from memory.

Asymmetries of the middle third are also often multifactorial. A septal deviation that was not causing asymmetry before dorsal reduction may become "unmasked" after dorsal reduction, and thereby cause asymmetries of the middle vault. Asymmetric dorsal reduction of the middle third can also occur. Palpation of the dorsum with moistened gloves allows careful assessment of the underlying anatomy after dorsal reduction.

Establishing symmetry at the tip is highly dynamic and requires an understanding of all major and minor tip support elements, as shown in **Table 1**.[1] Careful attention to tip suture technique and proper suture placement will help minimize tip asymmetries. Preexisting asymmetries of the medial and lateral crura may not be evident until other tip dynamics are altered. Similar to the middle third, a septal deviation that was not causing any asymmetry preoperatively may become "unmasked" as a result of

Disclosures: The authors have nothing to disclose.
Division of Facial Plastic and Reconstructive Surgery, Stanford Department of Otolaryngology/Head and Neck Surgery, 801 Welch Road, Stanford, CA 94305, USA
* Corresponding author.
E-mail address: jsurowitz@ohns.stanford.edu

Facial Plast Surg Clin N Am 21 (2013) 639–651
http://dx.doi.org/10.1016/j.fsc.2013.07.003
1064-7406/13/$ – see front matter © 2013 Elsevier Inc. All rights reserved.

Table 1
Complications of rhinoplasty

Complication	Cause	Avoidance	Correction
Asymmetry of the bony vault	Asymmetric osteotomies	Meticulous attention to osteotomies	Percutaneous osteotomies
Asymmetry of the middle vault	Unmasked dorsal septal deviation after dorsal reduction	Recognition of septal deviation	Crushed cartilage camouflage grafts
Tip asymmetry	Asymmetric tip sutures Unmasked caudal septal deviation	Meticulous attention to suture technique Meticulous inspection	Revision Possible placement of septal extension graft Possible repositioning of caudal septum with swinging door, secure to nasal spine with suture
Overresection of nasal bones	Overaggressive resection	Judicious bony dorsal reduction	Placement of dorsal onlay graft
Open roof deformity	Bony dorsal reduction	Judicious bony dorsal reduction when no osteotomies are planned, but unavoidable when narrowing of the bony base is planned	Lateral osteotomies to close open roof
Rocker deformity	Continuation of osteotomies into frontal bone	Meticulous planning of osteotomies and continuous palpation/inspection	Percutaneous osteotomies
Stair step deformity	Improper placement of lateral osteotomy anterior to the ascending process of the maxilla	Meticulous planning of osteotomies and continuous palpation/inspection	Percutaneous osteotomies
Pollybeak deformity	Overresection of nasal bones Underresection of dorsal septum (anterior septal angle) Postoperative soft tissue scar formation	Meticulous planning of dorsal reduction, both bony and cartilaginous dorsum Avoid overaggressive dorsal reduction in thick-skinned patients	Dorsal onlay camouflage graft Appropriately match cartilaginous dorsal reduction to that of bony dorsal reduction May require revision Kenalog injections postoperatively
Inverted V deformity	Upper lateral cartilages drop inferior and posterior, causing show of the nasal bones and dorsal septum This results from failure to repair the upper laterals to the dorsal septum after dorsal reduction	Repair upper lateral cartilages to dorsal septum after dorsal reduction Use of spreader grafts or autospreader grafts	Revision with use of spreader grafts (if upper lateral cartilage present), possible onlay crushed cartilage camouflage grafts, consider osteotomies to narrow the bony base if this is a contributing factor

Complication	Cause	Prevention	Treatment
Saddle nose deformity	Overaggressive dorsal reduction with septoplasty, resulting in a dorsal strut that is inadequate to support cartilaginous dorsum	Maintain 1.5-cm dorsal strut	Revision with dorsal onlay camouflage graft (minor cosmetic deformity) and rib cartilage graft reconstruction (severe cases)
Bossae	Overaggressive cephalic trim of lateral crura	Note predisposing factors for bossae formation (see below), avoid overaggressive resection	Revision with structural grafting of lateral crura (strut grafts), crushed cartilage, and/or temporalis fascia camouflage grafts
Visible grafts	Thin skin	Note thin skin preoperatively and place temporalis fascia overlay grafts to camouflage	Revision with possible graft removal and/or placement of temporalis fascia for contour smoothing and camouflage
Pinched tip	Overresection of lateral crura during cephalic trim	Spare 6- to 7-mm rim strip	Lateral crural strut grafts, possible crushed cartilage grafts for camouflage
	Malpositioning of lateral crura	Ensure appropriate orientation and positioning of lateral crura	Removal/revision of any offending tip sutures, possible lateral crural strut grafting, possible repositioning of lateral crura
	Contracture from wound healing		Revision surgery with one or more of the above maneuvers
Poorly defined tip	Overaggressive tip deprojection in thick-skinned patient	Avoid overaggressive deprojection	Judicious superficial nasalis aponeurotic system (SNAS) excision intraoperatively, Kenalog injections postoperatively
Nostril asymmetry	Altered caudal septum, medial, intermediate, and lateral crura dynamics from intraoperative suture technique or alteration	Meticulous attention to symmetric placement of sutures, such as tip and tongue in groove sutures	Revision, with correction of underlying offending cause
Alar retraction	Overly tight closure of marginal incision		Remove/revise offending sutures
	Overresection of lateral crura during cephalic trim		Lateral crural strut grafts, possible alar rim grafts (minor cases), auricular composite grafts (severe cases)
	Malpositioning of the lateral crura		Repositioning of the lateral crura, lateral crural strut grafts, possible alar rime grafts (minor cases), auricular composite grafts (severe cases)
	Overly tight lateral crural spanning sutures		Removal/revision of any offending tip sutures
	Contracture from wound healing		Revision surgery with one or more of the above maneuvers

(continued on next page)

Table 1
(continued)

Complication	Cause	Avoidance	Correction
Columellar retraction	Overresection of the caudal septum	Avoid overresection	Caudal septal extension graft, columellar strut graft, columellar plumping graft
	Excessive setback of the medial crura during tongue-in-groove	Avoid excessive setback	Revise tongue-in-groove, consider columellar plumping graft. Septocolumellar suture can be used to help prevent contracture during wound healing
Columellar and alar base scar formation	Wound healing	Meticulous wound closure	Kenalog injections with revision reserved for severe cases
Nasal obstruction	External nasal valve collapse	Maintain integrity and appropriate position of lateral crura, avoid overaggressive narrowing of the alar base	Lateral crural strut grafts, possible alar rim grafts
	Internal nasal valve collapse	Avoid overaggressive narrowing of the bony base, use spreader grafts or autospreader grafts to maintain patency	Spreader or autospreader grafts
	Septal deviation	Appropriately address any septal deviation	Septoplasty
	Intranasal synechia	Careful soft tissue handling and fastidious wound closure	Lysis of synechia
	Recurvature of the lateral crura	Recognize contribution to the patency of the nasal airway	Lateral crural strut grafts
Septal perforation	Opposing mucoperichondrial lacerations	Meticulous elevation of mucoperichondrial flaps to prevent opposing lacerations	Place fascia or crushed cartilage graft interposed between lacerations
	Septal hematoma	Placement of septal whip sutures and use of removable soft silastic intranasal splints, prophylactic mucoperichondrial flap incision to allow drainage of any accumulated blood	Incision and drainage
Costal cartilage (autograft and homograft) warping	Intrinsic property of cartilage	Concentric carving	Revision
Pneumothorax after costal cartilage harvest	Injury to the pleura	Harvest cartilage in subperichondrial plane	Close wound under water seal with positive pressure ventilation

surgical maneuvers, with resultant tip asymmetry or deviation. Contracture of the skin soft tissue envelope can also result in asymmetry of the tip over time.

Edema of the soft tissue envelope can make asymmetries and irregularities difficult to discern intraoperatively. Thus, careful marking before injection is paramount. Asymmetries can be minimized through judicious inspection from the top of the patient's head and through careful palpation using sterile saline-moistened gloves.

THE BONY PYRAMID
Overresection of the Nasal Bones

Overresection of the nasal bones can be avoided through judicious dorsal reduction, as seen in **Fig. 1**. Notice that this patient also has a pollybeak deformity, which is discussed later. More bone may easily be removed, whereas replacement after overresection presents a more challenging scenario.

Open Roof Deformity

An open roof is a normal consequence of dorsal reduction. Failure to close an open roof with appropriate osteotomies will result in a "flat top" appearance to the bony pyramid, as seen in **Fig. 2**. Edema of the soft tissue envelope can mask an open roof deformity on visual inspection.

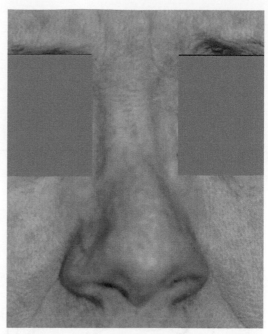

Fig. 2. Open roof deformity after prior rhinoplasty from failure to close with osteotomies.

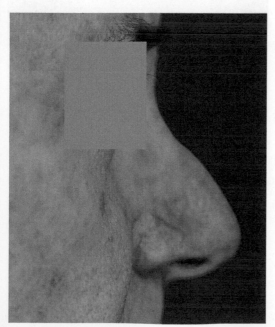

Fig. 1. Overresected nasal bones after prior rhinoplasty. Also note prominent pollybeak.

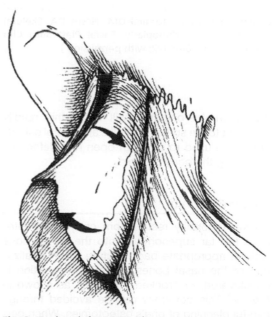

Fig. 3. Rocker deformity with osteotomies continuing into frontal gone. Note superior aspect "rocking" laterally when bony base is medialized. (*From* Toriumi DM, Hecht DA. Skeletal modifications in rhinoplasty. Facial Plast Surg Clin North Am 2000;8(4):424; with permission.)

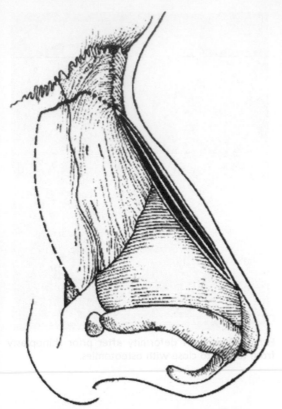

Fig. 4. Appropriate placement of osteotomies is demonstrated. Note lateral osteotomy in high-low-high fashion, fading medial osteotomy, with controlled back-fracture connecting medial and lateral osteotomies. (*From* Toriumi DM, Hecht DA. Skeletal modifications in rhinoplasty. Facial Plast Surg Clin North Am 2000;8(4):422; with permission.)

Again, careful palpation will make this readily apparent to the surgeon. Medial and lateral osteotomies are used to close an open roof deformity, narrowing the bony pyramid.

Rocker Deformity

Rocker deformity results from carrying osteotomies too far superiorly up into the frontal bone without appropriate back fracture. On medialization of the nasal bones, the superior portion is cantilevered, or "rocked," laterally, as shown in **Fig. 3.**[2] This deformity can be avoided through careful planning of one's osteotomies. When performing an endonasal lateral osteotomy, the guarded portion of the osteotome is oriented laterally and the surgeon continually palpates during the osteotomization process. Should this complication be encountered, transverse percutaneous

osteotomies may be performed to create the appropriate controlled back fracture.

Stair Step Deformity

Stair step deformity is caused by placement of the lateral osteotomy anterior to the ascending process of the maxilla, resulting in a palpable step-off. The lateral osteotomy should be placed along the ascending process (also known as the frontal process) of the maxilla in the standard high-low-high fashion, which is illustrated **Fig. 4.**[2] Careful planning of the lateral osteotomies will help the surgeon avoid this complication. The guarded portion of the osteotome is oriented laterally, and the surgeon continually palpates during the osteotomization process. In addition to careful palpation, the surgeon must listen for the distinct sound made when the osteotomy is being placed in the correct location along the ascending process of the maxilla. Percutaneous perforating lateral osteotomies also lend a degree of safety. This problem is difficult to correct, and therefore stair step deformity must be avoided.

THE MIDDLE THIRD
Pollybeak Deformity

Pollybeak deformity results when the lower third of the dorsum is more projected than the tip.

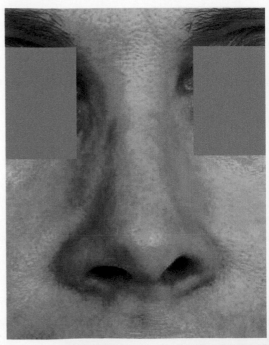

Fig. 5. Inverted V deformity is noted with prominence of the bony base and narrowing of the middle third.

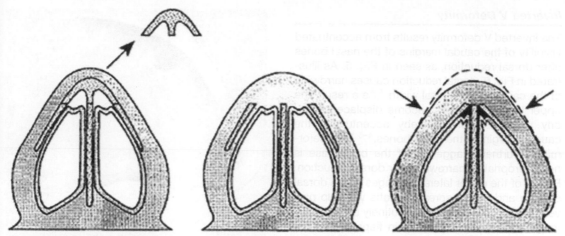

Fig. 6. Noted dorsal narrowing after cartilaginous dorsal reduction. (*From* Toriumi DM. Management of the middle nasal vault in rhinoplasty. Facial Plast Surg Clin North Am 1995;2(1):18; with permission.)

This is seen in **Fig. 1.** Overresection of the bony pyramid, underresection of the cartilaginous middle third (specifically the anterior septal angle), and supratip fibrosis deep to the soft tissue envelope can all result in pollybeak.[1] The first 2 are preventable, whereas the third occurs postoperatively in the setting of wound healing. Additionally, loss of tip support with subsequent tip ptosis can result in a relative pollybeak. Palpation allows the surgeon to assess the dorsum and to

determine if additional resection is necessary. Soft tissue pollybeak can be addressed with Kenalog injections to the affected area. The senior author prefers to use a very conservative Kenalog 10 mixed 1:10 or 1:5 with 1% lidocaine with 1:100,000 epinephrine. It is critical that all Kenalog be injected deep to the dermis to avoid dermal thinning. Overaggressive injection can itself cause divots from dermal or cartilaginous injury.

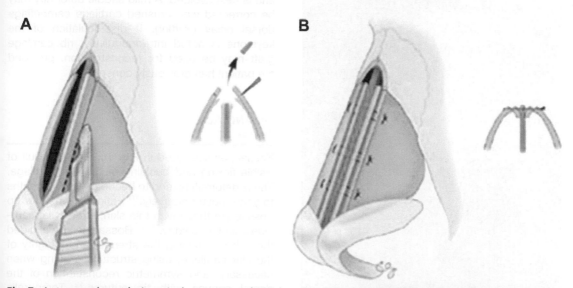

Fig. 7. Autospreader technique is shown. Upper lateral cartilage is scored (*A*), subsequently folded on itself and suture repaired to the dorsal septum (*B*). (*From* Yoo S, Most SP. Nasal airway preservation using the autospreader technique: analysis of outcomes using a disease-specific quality-of-life instrument. Arch Facial Plast Surg 2011;13(4):232; with permission.)

Inverted V Deformity

The inverted V deformity results from accentuated visibility of the caudal margins of the nasal bones after dorsal reduction, as seen in **Fig. 5**. As illustrated in **Fig. 6**, dorsal reduction causes narrowing of the cartilaginous dorsal width.[3] As a result, the upper lateral cartilages become displaced inferiorly and posteriorly, thereby accentuating the caudal margin of the nasal bones.[4–6] This deformity is further exaggerated if the bony base is not appropriately narrowed after dorsal reduction. Repair of the upper lateral cartilages to the dorsal septum and use of spreader grafts will help prevent this.[6] The senior author routinely uses the autospreader upper lateral turn-in flaps, which are shown in **Fig. 7**.[7]

Saddle Nose Deformity

The saddle nose deformity may be the result of overresection of the quadrangular cartilage with insufficient dorsal strut. A postoperative saddle deformity is seen in **Fig. 8**. Inadvertent disarticulation of the keystone area, in which the quadrangular cartilage fuses superiorly with the perpendicular plate of the ethmoid, may also result

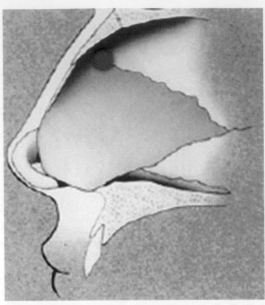

Fig. 9. The keystone area is highlighted in red. (*From* Tardy ME, Toriumi DM Jr, Hecht DA. Functional and aesthetic surgery of the nose. In: Papel ID, editor. Facial plastic and reconstructive surgery. 2nd edition. Thieme; New York: 2002. p. 370; with permission.)

in saddling. The keystone is shown in **Fig. 9**.[8] Extracorporeal septoplasty is particularly prone to this and can be avoided using the anterior septal reconstruction technique.[9]

Saddle nose deformity can be difficult to correct and is best avoided. A mild saddle deformity may be corrected with crushed cartilage camouflage dorsal onlay grafting. If disarticulation of the keystone is noted intraoperatively, rib cartilage graft may be used for reconstruction, provided the patient has previously consented.

TIP AND ALA
Bossae

Bossae, as illustrated in **Fig. 10**, are the result of visible flexing and buckling of the alar cartilage. These deformities tend to become evident months to years postoperatively.[10] Patients at risk for tip bossae are those with thin skin, strong alar cartilages, and tip bifidity.[10,11] Bossae can be avoided through maintaining the strength and integrity of the alar cartilage, using structural grafting when necessary, and symmetric reconstitution of the domal subunit with tip sutures.[12] Temporalis fascia or crushed cartilage may also be used in thin-skinned patients to help camouflage any irregularities.

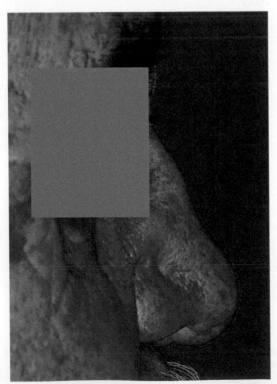

Fig. 8. Saddle nose deformity after prior rhinoplasty.

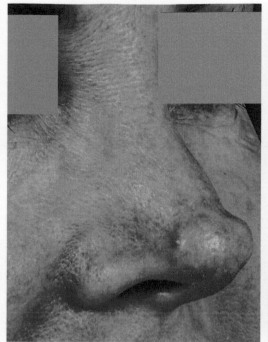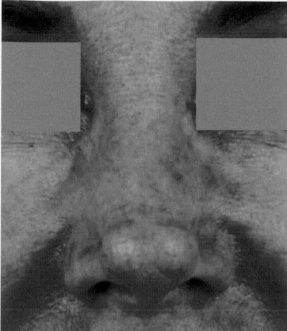

Fig. 10. Bossae are seen after prior rhinoplasty.

Visible Grafts

In thin-skinned individuals, tip grafts can become visible over time as the skin soft tissue envelope contracts and thins. Therefore, avoiding tip grafts in very thin-skinned individuals is preferable, because this complication is often noted at a later date, after edema has decreased and the skin soft tissue envelope has begun contracting, and must be addressed with formal revision. The authors often use temporalis fascia as a camouflage graft in thin-skinned patients if grafts must be used.

Pinched Tip

A pinched tip may result from overaggressive cephalic resection of the lateral crura, which results in weakening of the remaining rim strip (**Fig. 11**).[13] Care must be taken to avoid overresection during cephalic trim. The senior author preserves at least a 7-mm rim strip to avoid overresection during cephalic trim. Malpositioning of the lateral crura, with the caudal border placed significantly inferior to the cephalic border, may similarly result in a pinched tip, as described by Toriumi and Checcone[14,15] and illustrated in **Fig. 12**. Lateral crural repositioning and lateral crural strut grafts may be used to facilitate appropriate orientation of the lateral crura.[14–16]

Poorly Defined Tip

The poorly defined or amorphous tip can occur in thick-skinned individuals after tip deprojection and suture modification. Recognizing thick skin preoperatively and avoiding overaggressive deprojection in thick-skinned individuals is key. Judicious SNAS excision may be performed to help improve tip definition.

Nostril Asymmetries

Nostril asymmetries can occur from an unmasked septal deviation after caudal septal resection,

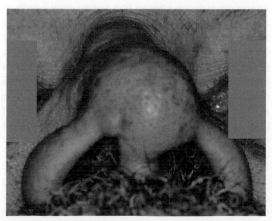

Fig. 11. Pinched tip after prior rhinoplasty.

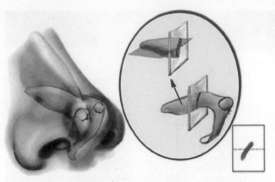

Fig. 12. Pinched tip may result from malpositioned lateral crura, with caudal margin positioned significantly inferior to cephalic margin. (*From* Toriumi DM. New concepts in nasal tip contouring. Arch Facial Plast Surg 2006;8(3):162; with permission.)

placement of a septal extension graft, or asymmetric tip modifications. It is important to recognize any preoperative nostril asymmetries and counsel patients appropriately in this regard. The authors routinely perform a nostril check before final closure to ensure appropriate symmetry.

Alar-Columellar Disproportion

Gunter and Friedman[16] previously described the alar-columellar relationship and classification of related deformities. This article focuses on alar retraction, columellar retraction, and hanging columella. **Fig. 13** shows both alar retraction and a hanging columella.

Alar retraction may result from overly tight closure of marginal incisions, especially as one approaches the nasal facets. Careful attention to closure of the marginal incisions can help avoid Alar retraction. Overaggressive resection during cephalic trim can result in contracture of the lateral crura superiorly with time and wound healing, thereby causing alar retraction.[17] Lateral crural spanning sutures placed too tightly may result in alar retraction.[18] The orientation of the lateral crura is also of importance. As described by Toriumi and Checcone,[15] the caudal margin of the lateral crura should lie in a plane almost horizontal and oriented just inferior to the cephalic margin. This technique prevents cephalic positioning of the lateral crura and helps support the alar rim. Alar retraction may be corrected with the use of alar rim grafts in minor cases (**Fig. 14**), with placement of ear composite grafts in more severe cases (**Fig. 15**).[17]

Columellar retraction may result from overaggressive resection of the caudal septum, medial crura, or excessive setback of the medial crura after placement of a tongue-in-groove suture.[17] An overly resected caudal septum may be addressed

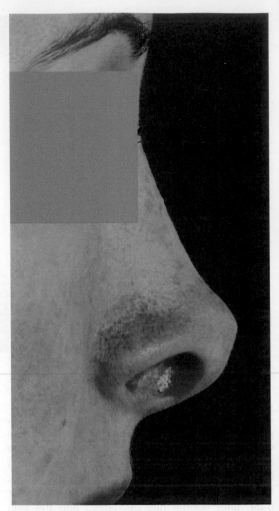

Fig. 13. Patient with both alar retraction and hanging columella after previous rhinoplasty.

with a caudal septal extension graft with or without tongue-in-groove repair of the medial crural footplates. Excessive setback after tongue-in-groove suture is best addressed through revision of the tongue-in-groove until the desired effect is achieved. Columellar struts or plumping grafts may also be helpful adjunctive measures in certain cases.

A hanging columella may result from placement of an overly large columellar strut graft, septal extension graft, or tip graft.[17] Contributing anatomy includes the caudal septum, medial crura, intermediate crura, and membranous septum. Tip deprojection and decreased rotation may also contribute.[17] Depending on the origin, a hanging columella can be addressed by selective resection of the caudal septum and tongue-in-groove suture technique.

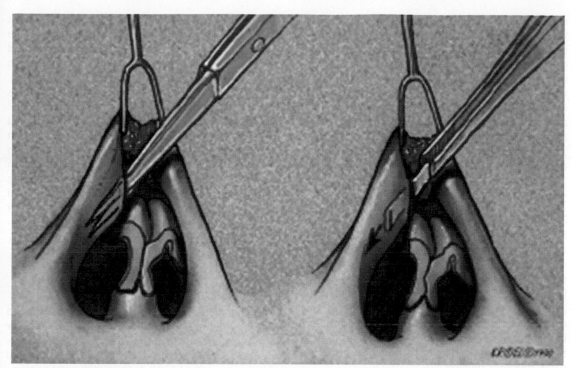

Fig. 14. Placement of alar rim grafts. (*From* Kridel RW, Chiu RJ. The management of alar columellar disproportion in revision rhinoplasty. Facial Plast Surg Clin North Am 2006;14(4):326; with permission.)

COLUMELLA AND ALAR BASE
Scar Formation

Patients should be counseled about the potential for scar formation from the columellar incision in external rhinoplasty and with all alar base excisions. Unsightly columellar scars, hypertrophic scars, and keloids are very uncommon. Alar base excisions put the patient at risk for visible scar formation. The columellar incision is performed using an inverted V, so as to prevent scar formation.[19]

Meticulous attention to closure will help prevent columellar and alar base scar formation.

AIRWAY

Nasal obstruction can occur as a result of external nasal valve collapse, internal nasal valve collapse, septal deviation, and intranasal synechia formation. Weak lateral crura can be reinforced with lateral crural strut grafts.[16] Spreader grafts may be used to widen the patency of the internal nasal

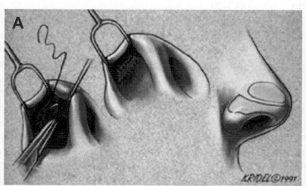

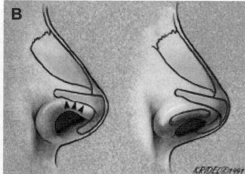

Fig. 15. Auricular composite grafts may be used to address alar retraction. These grafts may be placed at the level of the scroll (*A*) or at the caudal margin of the lateral crura (*B*). (*From* Kridel RW, Chiu RJ. The management of alar columellar disproportion in revision rhinoplasty. Facial Plast Surg Clin North Am 2006;14(4):319; with permission.)

valve.[5,6,20,21] The senior author routinely uses autospreaders, as previously noted and illustrated in **Fig. 7**.[7] Meticulous inspection of nostril symmetry, position of the caudal septum, and an understanding of the dynamics of the internal nasal valve will help minimize postoperative nasal obstruction. Recurvature of the lateral crura may also result in nasal airway obstruction, especially after maneuvers that narrow the nasal base, such as alar base excisions. Lateral crural strut grafts can be used to mitigate recurvature.

SEPTUM

Septal Perforation

Septal perforation is a known risk of any septal surgery and patients should be counseled in this regard. Prior septoplasty places the patient at a higher risk. Meticulous dissection of the mucoperichondrial flaps, with avoidance of lacerating the mucosa on both sides directly opposing one another will help minimize the risk of perforation. If bilateral opposing perforations occur intraoperatively, a crushed cartilage graft may be placed to allow mucosal healing.

Septal Hematoma

A septal hematoma is a risk of any septal surgery. These complications result when blood accumulates within any dead space between the elevated mucoperichondrial flaps. Septal hematomas predispose patients to infection and septal perforation. Use of transseptal whip sutures, placement of inferiorly based drainage incisions, and use of soft silastic removable intranasal splints will help minimize hematoma formation. Once a hematoma develops, it should be drained immediately.

COSTAL CARTILAGE GRAFTS

Costal cartilage grafts, including autologous and homologous, may become visible from warping over time. This deformity occurs from the intrinsic properties of cartilage. Concentric carving can mitigate this to some degree, but it is important to counsel patients regarding the risk of cartilage warping and subsequent irregularities or visibility of the graft.

Pneumothorax is a rare complication from autologous cartilage harvest. The risk of this is roughly 1% and can usually be managed without a chest tube. Should the surgeon encounter a pneumothorax, the injury is usually confined to the parietal pleura.[22] Management consists of inserting a sterile red rubber catheter into the wound, placing the distal end of the catheter into sterile saline (as a water seal). Anesthesia then administers positive

pressure ventilation and the wound is closed as the catheter is removed. Patients should receive a postoperative chest radiograph and be admitted for observation, with a repeat chest radiograph on the morning of postoperative day one.

Homograft costal cartilage has a theoretical risk of resorption over time. Kridel and colleagues[23] found no significant difference between autologous and homologous cartilage with regard to resorption or infection. The senior author has been using homologous costal cartilage with good results in patients who are not candidates for autologous grafts because of age (ossification), severity of obstructive sleep apnea, other comorbidities, or patient preference. It is important to counsel patients regarding the theoretical risk of resorption, although this does not seem to manifest clinically.

SUMMARY

The dynamics of nasal aesthetics and function are very complex, and therefore the potential for complications are myriad. A thorough understanding of nasal anatomy and how various surgical maneuvers affect both form and function is imperative. Certain complications are within the surgeon's control, such as those related to technique, whereas those related to patient wound healing are out of the surgeon's control. Careful patient selection, history, physical examination, photo documentation, and patient counseling about appropriate expectations are important aspects of the surgery and should not be underestimated.

REFERENCES

1. Tardy ME Jr, Kron TK, Younger R, et al. The cartilaginous pollybeak: etiology, prevention, and treatment. Facial Plast Surg 1989;6(2):113–20.
2. Toriumi DM, Hecht DA. Skeletal modifications in rhinoplasty. Facial Plast Surg Clin North Am 2000;8(4): 413–30.
3. Toriumi DM. Management of the middle nasal vault in rhinoplasty. Facial Plast Surg Clin North Am 1995;2(1):18.
4. Constantian MB. The incompetent external nasal valve: pathophysiology and treatment in primary and secondary rhinoplasty. Plast Reconstr Surg 1994;93(5):919–31 [discussion: 932–3].
5. Rohrich RJ, Hollier LH. Use of spreader grafts in the external approach to rhinoplasty. Clin Plast Surg 1996;23(2):255–62.
6. Sheen JH. Spreader graft: a method of reconstructing the roof of the middle nasal vault following rhinoplasty. Plast Reconstr Surg 1984;73(2):230–9.
7. Yoo S, Most SP. Nasal airway preservation using the autospreader technique: analysis of outcomes using

a disease-specific quality-of-life instrument. Arch Facial Plast Surg 2011;13(4):231–3.

8. Tardy ME Jr, Toriumi DM, Hecht DA. Functional and aesthetic surgery of the nose. In: Papel ID, editor. Facial plastic and reconstructive surgery. 2nd edition. New York: Thieme; 2002. p. 370.

9. Most SP. Anterior septal reconstruction: outcomes after a modified extracorporeal septoplasty technique. Arch Facial Plast Surg 2006;8(3):202–7.

10. Kridel R, Yoon P, Koch R. Prevention and correction of nasal tip bossae in rhinoplasty. Arch Facial Plast Surg 2003;5(5):416–22.

11. Gillman G, Simons R, Lee D. Nasal tip bossae in rhinoplasty. Etiology, predisposing factors, and management techniques. Arch Facial Plast Surg 1999; 1(2):83–9.

12. Brenner M, Hilger P. Thin skin rhinoplasty: aesthetic considerations and surgical approach. In: Azizzadeh B, Murphy MR, Johnson CM, et al, editors. Master techniques in rhinoplasty. Philadelphia: Elsevier; 2011. p. 331–4.

13. Paun S, Trenite G. Correction of the pinched nasal tip deformity. In: Azizzadeh B, Murphy MR, Johnson CM, et al, editors. Master techniques in rhinoplasty. Philadelphia: Elsevier; 2011. p. 235–44.

14. Toriumi DM. New concepts in nasal tip contouring. Arch Facial Plast Surg 2006;8(3):156–85.

15. Toriumi DM, Checcone MA. New concepts in nasal tip contouring. Facial Plast Surg Clin North Am 2009;17(1):55–90, vi.

16. Gunter JP, Friedman RM. Lateral crural strut graft: technique and clinical applications in rhinoplasty. Plast Reconstr Surg 1997;99(4):943–52 [discussion: 953–5].

17. Kridel RW, Chiu. The management of alar columellar disproportion in revision rhinoplasty. Facial Plast Surg Clin North Am 2006;14(4):313–29, vi.

18. Baker S. Suture contouring of the nasal tip. Arch Facial Plast Surg 2000;2(1):34–42.

19. Davis RE. Proper execution of the transcolumellar incision in external rhinoplasty. Ear Nose Throat J 2004;83(4):232–3.

20. Most SP. Trends in functional rhinoplasty. Arch Facial Plast Surg 2008;10(6):410–3.

21. Most SP. Analysis of outcomes after functional rhinoplasty using a disease-specific quality-of-life instrument. Arch Facial Plast Surg 2006;8(5):306–9.

22. Marin VP, Landecker A, Gunter JP. Harvesting rib cartilage grafts for secondary rhinoplasty. Plast Reconstr Surg 2008;121(4):1442–8.

23. Kridel RW, Ashoori F, Liu ES, et al. Long-term use and follow-up of irradiated homologous costal cartilage grafts in the nose. Arch Facial Plast Surg 2009; 11(6):378–94.

Complications of Otoplasty

Ethan B. Handler, MD, Tara Song, MD, Charles Shih, MD*

KEYWORDS

- Otoplasty • Complications • Protruding ears • Prominent ears • Treatment

KEY POINTS

- Do not overtighten antihelix horizontal mattress sutures to avoid the hidden helix.
- Take full-thickness cartilage bites including the anterior perichondrium to avoid cartilage pull-through of mattress sutures and relapse.
- Avoid external canal narrowing by placing posteriorly oriented concha-mastoid sutures or excising cartilage.
- Cartilage splitting or scoring techniques run the risk of visible cartilage irregularities or sharp edges.
- Do not rely on skin excision to hold ear position.

INTRODUCTION

Auricular proportions and defining characteristics of the pinna have been well documented and defined in the literature. Although the function of the pinna in regards to hearing is minor, the social and psychological impact of having protruding or prominent ears is profound. This anatomic variation occurs in approximately 5% of the population, and usually by school age, children become very self-conscious of their "Dumbo or mouse ears." Correcting this deformity can help children gain self-esteem and prevent social ridicule.[1]

The earliest auricular surgery dates back to seventh century in the writings of Sushruta, an Indian healer whose teachings were rooted in Ayurveda.[2] In 1848, JF Dieffenbach published a novel otoplasty technique using sutures to pin the ears back through an incision made in the post-auricular sulcus.[3] Otoplasty surgery is usually directed toward 2 specific areas, the conchal bowl, which is often hypertrophied, and the antihelix, which may be flattened and/or underdeveloped, or a combination of both. The aesthetically pleasing auricle projects approximately 20° to 30° from the skull (**Fig. 1**). The length of the ear is approximately 55 to 60 mm when fully developed, and the width is approximately 55% of the length. Furthermore, along its vertical axis, the auricle sits a gentle 20° posterior.[4]

One of the better objective measurements is the helical to scalp distance, which is measured at 3 points, the superior point of the helical rim, the midpoint of the helix, and the lobule (**Fig. 2**). These distances range from 10 to 12 mm, 16 to 20 mm, and 20 to 22 mm, respectively. In bilateral otoplasty, these measurements serve as a guide for the surgeon, and documentation of these distances is important in creating symmetry. In the unilateral otoplasty, measurements from the aesthetically better ear can be used to gauge setback of the protruding one.[5]

Currently, 2 schools of thought predominate regarding otoplastic surgery summarized broadly as cartilage cutting and cartilage sparing techniques. The former involves removal of cartilage and the scoring of cartilage, whereas the latter involves contouring by placement of either permanent or absorbable sutures. Cartilage cutting techniques tend to be favored in Europe and are liked due to the durability of the correction over time, although there exists a higher risk of anterior cartilage irregularities.[6] Typically, the otoplasty is

The authors have nothing to disclose.
Department of Head and Neck Surgery, Kaiser Permanente Medical Center, 280 West MacArthur Boulevard, Oakland, CA 94611, USA
* Corresponding author.
E-mail address: charles.shih@kp.org

facialplastic.theclinics.com

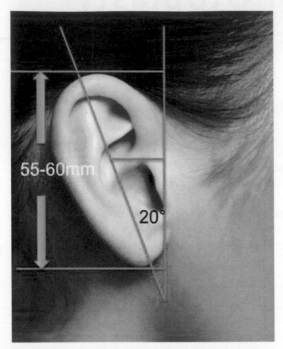

Fig. 1. Normal ear is oriented approximately 20° posterior from the vertical axis. The length of the adult ear is approximately 55 to 60 mm, the width approximately 55% of the length.

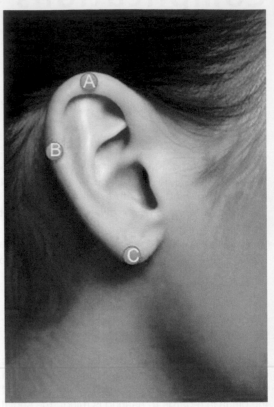

Fig. 2. Distances from points A, B, C to the underlying scalp are 10 to 12 mm, 16 to 20 mm, and 20 to 22 mm respectively. These distances help the surgeon standardize measurements from the unaffected ear to the protruding one or with bilateral otoplasty surgery.

performed with wedge excisions, scoring, abrasion, and cartilaginous incisions on either the anterior or the posterior cartilage surface in an attempt to counteract the spring of the unfurled antihelix. In North America, cartilage sparing techniques predominate, namely the Furnas[7] and the Mustarde,[8] or variations on these techniques. The advantages include less scaring, allowance of easy suture adjustment, preservation of the cartilage framework, and prevention of contour irregularities. Where it may fall short is with stability of the operation over time.[9]

Fortunately, complications of otoplasty are relatively uncommon and can usually be avoided with meticulous preoperative, intraoperative, and postoperative care from both the patient and surgeon perspective. The surgeon must be familiar with the range of complications and must appropriately counsel the patient before surgery about these risks, in addition to being ready to confidently handle them if they arise. The cumulative rate of early complication has been cited from 0% to 8.4%, with information on late complications varying greatly between 0% and 47.3%.[10] Granted, the literature is varied and most studies are retrospective reviews of surgical cases for individual institutions or surgeons. Most important to the otoplastic surgeon is a depth of understanding of the various

techniques and complications so that the best result is obtained (**Table 1**).

EARLY COMPLICATIONS

These complications typically occur within hours to days after the procedure.

Post-operative Hematoma/Hemorrhage

The external ear is supplied by multiple arterial sources. This extensive vasculature makes it a resilient candidate for multiple surgical approaches (**Fig. 3**). The blood supply to the external ear is derived mainly from branches of the external carotid artery, namely the superficial temporal artery and the posterior auricular artery.[11]

To minimize intraoperative bleeding, the skin should be injected with 1% lidocaine with 1:100,000 epinephrine before incision. During the procedure, great care should be taken to respect tissue planes as well as maintain hemostasis, preferably with bipolar electrocautery.

Table 1
Otoplasty complications

Early	Late
Hematoma	Hypertrophic scar/keloids
Infection/ Perichondritis	Suture complications
Cartilage/Skin necrosis	Recurrence
	• Auricular deformities
	○ Telephone ear/reverse telephone ear
	○ Vertical post-deformity
	○ Overcorrection helix
	○ Hidden helix
	○ Auricular ridges
	○ Antihelical malposition/ puckering
	○ Narrowing external auditory canal meatus

Bleeding can occur post-operatively once the vasoconstrictive effects of the local anesthetic have worn off, if appropriate hemostasis is not achieved before closure or if post-operative trauma occurs. Occult coagulopathies will ideally be identified preoperatively with a thorough history and physical exam. One of the hallmark signs of post-operative hematoma is intense pain, which is especially concerning if it presents in a unilateral or asymmetric fashion. This should be managed with immediate exploration with the goal of evacuating the hematoma and achieving hemostasis to avoid complications of wound infection, perichondritis, or chondritis, all of which can lead to devastating anatomic deformity or "cauliflower ear."[12]

A compressive dressing may also be applied at the end of the operation to aid in prevention of hematoma. The authors' preferred choice of dressing is placement of xeroform into the concha and within the helix so that it is well formed in the crevices of the ear. Next, a Glasscock dressing is applied with a few of the fluffs removed as to not add too much pressure to the ear than may result in necrosis. This dressing is left on for 2 days, after which a headband is then worn continuously for 3 weeks.

Infection

Infection after otoplasty shares a common temporal trend with many surgical sites, typically manifesting after 3 to 4 days (**Fig. 4**). The incidence of infection is between 2.4% and 5.2%.[13] Appropriate preoperative sterile preparation and administration of peri-operative intravenous antibiotics, sterile and meticulous intraoperative surgical technique, and use of post-operative antibiotic ointment can all help to reduce the risk of post-operative infection.

Infection typically presents as visible erythema, edema or asymmetry, or drainage, or the patient

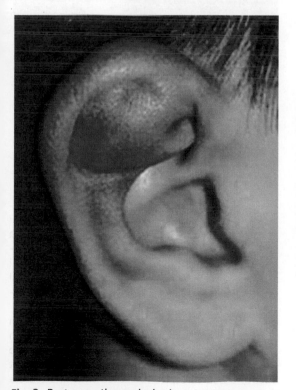

Fig. 3. Post-operative auricular hematoma.

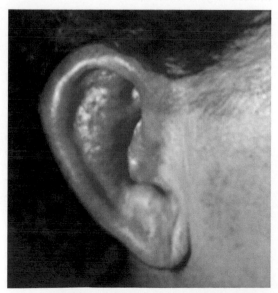

Fig. 4. Inflammation and erythema characteristic of perichondritis.

may complain of disproportionate amounts of pain relative to physical examination findings. The spectrum of infection may range from simple cellulitis to more extensive infection such as perichondritis or chondritis, the latter of which can lead to significant deformity of the auricle. Infection warrants drainage and administration of parenteral antibiotics to cover both *Pseudomonas Aeruginosa* and gram-positive organisms. Tissue debridement may also be necessary if necrosis has occurred.[14]

Skin and Cartilage Necrosis

Cartilage necrosis will often occur as a result of an infection and will manifest as perichondritis. This often results in auricular deformity and may necessitate removal of the necrotic cartilage to remove the nidus of infection and prevent worsening auricular deformity. Skin necrosis is typically a result of flawed surgical technique and rough handling of the soft tissue and skin. The most likely factors are excessive cautery, poor surgical dissection, violation of the subdermal plexus blood supply, and excessively tight dressings. Pain that is disproportionate to the procedure is the most common complaint, and management is similar to hematoma with the addition of possible skin grafting needed if too much cartilage is exposed.[9]

LATE COMPLICATIONS

Late complications typically occur weeks to months after the procedure. They are usually more gradual in onset and can be overlooked without diligent follow-up.

Keloid and Hypertrophic Scarring

Certain individuals are predisposed to hypertrophic scarring, especially those with darker skin pigmentation and a personal or family history of hypertrophic scarring. Appropriate preoperative counseling should be undertaken to inform all patients about the risks of scarring. Nevertheless, planning incisions with care, minimizing tension at closure, and prevention of infection can help to avoid this complication. If keloids occur, they should be treated as they typically are at any other location. Intralesional triamcinolone (40 mg/mL) injection may be used to reduce the volume of hypertrophy, although more severe or refractory scarring may require excision, radiation, or pressure dressings.[15] If triamcinolone is used, patients should be counseled about the risks of intralesional injection including pain, hyperpigmentation or hypopigmentation of overlying skin, and tissue atrophy.

SUTURE COMPLICATIONS

There is a range of suture complications related to otoplasty, and the nature of the complication is primarily dependent on the type of suture used.

Commonly used techniques, such as those described by Furnas and Mustarde, use nonabsorbable sutures to sculpt a new antihelical fold and decrease the prominence of the conchal bowl. The use of both braided and monofilament sutures have been described, and each comes with drawbacks. Braided or polyfilament sutures tend to be more reactive and more commonly result in infection and granuloma formation (Fig. 5). Although less erosive than polyfilament, monofilament sutures such as prolene and nylon have the risk of eroding through the skin or causing a bowstringing appearance in the post-auricular sulcus underneath the thin skin. They also have the tendency to slip, which can result in malposition of the pinna.

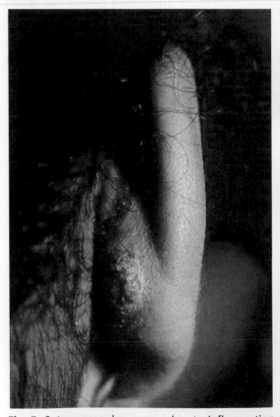

Fig. 5. Suture granuloma secondary to inflammation from the suture knot. Skin is usually friable and the wound easily entered. The knot is grasped with a smooth adson forceps and excised with fine scissors that may result in relapse.

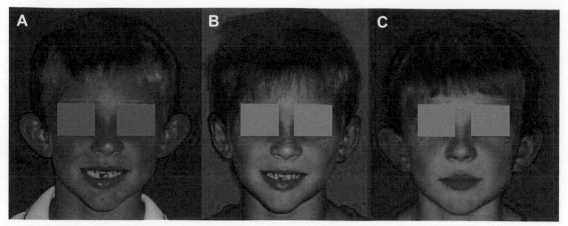

Fig. 6. Recurrence: (*A*) Pre-operative photographs; (*B*) 2 months post-op; (*C*) 6 months post op.

If infection or granuloma occurs, the timing of suture removal can be important in terms of cosmesis and maintenance of pinna position. If infection is indolent, removal can be delayed several months to allow time for further healing and expected scaring of soft tissues to avoid relapse of the initial malposition.

Hypoesthesia

The great auricular nerve is responsible for much of the sensory innervation to the external ear. Injury to the nerve or its small branches during otoplasty can result in sensory deficits or paresthesias. Most of these deficits will improve and resolve with time alone, although rare permanent

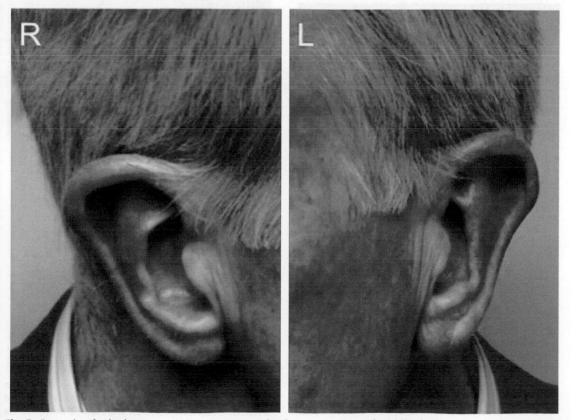

Fig. 7. Example of telephone ear deformity as a result of overcorrection of middle third portion of ear and over-resection of conchal bowl.

sensory complications have been reported. Patients have also reported decreased sensitivity to temperature, and this can be problematic in cold weather as patients are more susceptible to frostbite. Patients should be counseled to take appropriate precautions as needed.

Loss of Correction

This complication is one of the more common, ranging between 6.5% and 12%. Loss of correction is most affected by the type of technique used to correct the protruding ears (**Fig. 6**). Cartilage sparing techniques will have a higher rate of recurrence as compared with the cartilage cutting/contouring techniques. Skin-only excision as a means for setback will have the highest rate of recurrence. Furthermore, improper placement of sutures, placement of too few sutures causing increased tension and a "cheese wire" effect through the cartilage, and failure to overcorrect at the time surgery also contribute to recurrence. Mattress sutures placement should include a full-thickness cartilage bite through the anterior perichondrium. Improper placement may also lead to

the "cheese wire" effect through the cartilage. Some patients may have resilient cartilage with a strong intrinsic memory. Failure to address this with additional techniques such as scoring may contribute to loss of correction within a few months time. Lastly, post-operative trauma may cause sutures to pull through and disrupt the healing process.[16] Our typical post-operative dressing includes a sports headband at all times for the first 3 weeks, then a headband every night while sleeping for 3 additional weeks. Patients, especially children are cautioned about rough housing and contact activities. It is fairly common to elicit a history of trauma in children after seeing some loss of correction.

Patient Dissatisfaction

As with any operative procedure, appropriate patient selection and preoperative counseling is

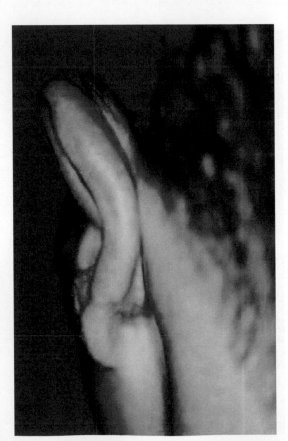

Fig. 8. Obliteration of sulcus from over resection of skin and conchal bowl cartilage.

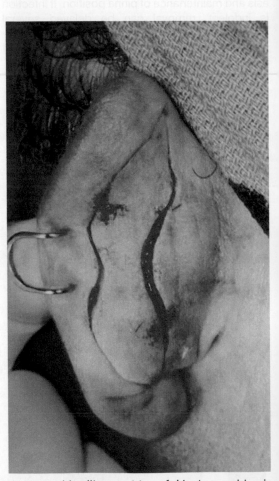

Fig. 9. Double ellipse excision of skin. Less excision in the mid-portion decreases risk of overcorrection and telephone ear. Skin excision should not be relied on to hold the desired contour. Cartilage needs to be adequately contoured to maintain shape.

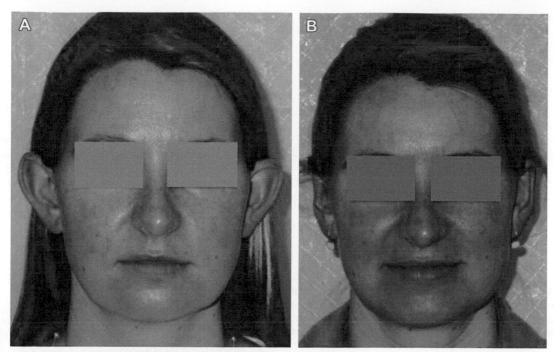

Fig. 10. Preop (*A*) and post-op (*B*) photographs showing overcorrection of right ear with hidden helix from prominent antihelix; this results from too much tightening with the Mustarde sutures.

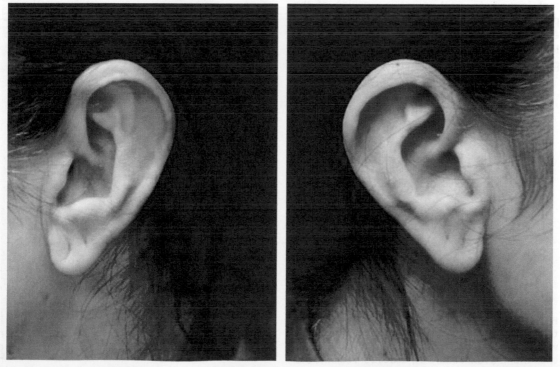

Fig. 11. Antihelical ridges secondary to cartilage-scoring technique. This patient had operation 20 years ago abroad.

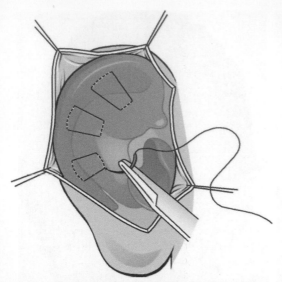

Fig. 12. Shows appropriate placement of horizontal mattress sutures. The superior most mattress suture must be oriented in a more vertical manner to prevent vertical post-deformity and to mimic the curve of the helix. (*Courtesy of* Andreas Naumann, MD, Munich, Germany.)

essential for setting patient expectations. A thorough explanation of risks of the procedure must be accompanied by a discussion about the fact that immediate post-operative position of the pinna may not be maintained and that additional efforts (including reoperation) may be necessary to achieve the desired result. A review of possible complications should be addressed.

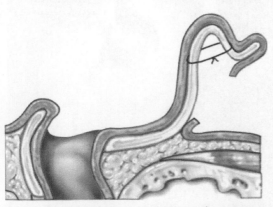

Fig. 13. Example of Mustarde horizontal mattress sutures. Notice the stitch when placed appropriately will be full thickness through the cartilage and perichondrium. (*From* Ambro BT, Lebeau J. Pediatric otoplasty. Operat Tech Otolaryngol Head Neck Surg 2009;20(3):208; with permission.)

TECHNICAL COMPLICATIONS
Telephone Ear Deformity/Reverse Telephone Ear Deformity

Telephone ear deformity occurs with overcorrection of the middle third of the ear excessively tightened with mattress sutures and/or overresection of the conchal bowl (**Fig. 7**). Overresection of the post-auricular skin can also contribute to telephone ear. Unrecognized lobular hypertrophy at the time of surgery may also contribute to the telephone ear. Reverse telephone ear is the opposite of the above, caused by overcorrection of the upper and lower one-third of the ear or under correction of the middle third.[15]

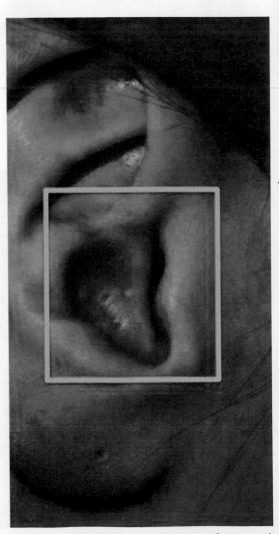

Fig. 14. A narrow external auditory canal as a result of a misplaced concha-mastoid suture.

Vertical Post-deformity

Vertical post-deformity occurs with careless placement of superior Mustarde mattress suture creating a vertically oriented superior crus rather than a gentle curvilinear arc that mimics the shape of the helix. This deformity is a complication that can be seen with direct visualization at the time of surgery and thus should be avoided intraoperatively.

Overcorrection and the Hidden Helix

When excessive conchal resection occurs along with excessive post-auricular skin removal, the ear can often have a stuck down appearance with obliteration of the post-auricular sulcus (**Figs. 8–10**). A dumbbell-shaped excision of skin is used to avoid excess excision at the middle third of the ear. The hidden helix occurs when the antihelix is overcorrected, and this will cause the antihelix to obscure the helix from frontal view when in actuality; the aesthetically pleasing contour is for the helix to be visible by a few millimeters from the frontal view.

Auricular Ridges

Auricular ridges are most often encountered with cartilage scoring or excision and will give a sharp-edged or jagged appearance of the antihelix (**Fig. 11**). These cartilage-cutting techniques can destabilize the auricular cartilage, and with new tensional forces during the healing period, can result in noticeable step-offs. These more aggressive techniques should be reserved for the particularly stiff cartilages and should be exercised with caution.

Antihelical Malposition/Puckering

The esthetic antihelix has a gentle curve and recreating this element in the protruding ear is paramount for a good outcome (**Figs. 12 and 13**). Positioning of the Mustarde mattress sutures should be parallel to the cartilage and perichondrium, staying subdermal, and be positioned at least 7 mm apart to not create too sharp of a fold. The exact position of sutures is marked on the ear before prepping the skin with a marker, then with a needle dipped in methylene blue to

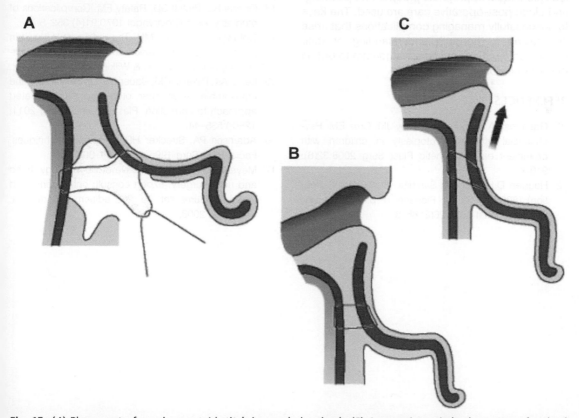

Fig. 15. (*A*) Placement of concha-mastoid stitch in conchal setback. (*B*) Appropriate stitch placement of setback stitch that keeps lateral external auditory canal (EAC) patent. (*C*) Malposition of stitch causing anterior displacement of concha, obscuring lateral EAC. (*Courtesy of* Andreas Naumann, MD, Munich, Germany.)

mark the underlying cartilage; this assures exact placement after the skin has been elevated from the cartilage post-auricularly.

Narrowing of External Auditory Canal Meatus

Iatrogenic meatal stenosis is a serious complication of otoplasty and is more common in adults as their cartilage tends to be thicker and less compliant (**Figs. 14** and **15**). Narrowing of the canal can result from overrotation of the conchal bowl when setback sutures are placed. Concha-mastoid sutures should be placed so the concha is pulled posteriorly to avoid narrowing the canal. In addition, cartilage is shaved from the posterior aspect of the conchal cartilage behind the external auditory canal, which also helps to facilitate retro displacement of the ear. If this complication is encountered, excision of excessive cartilage from an anterior or posterior approach is required to restore patency of the canal.[17]

SUMMARY

Fortunately, complications after otoplasty are relatively uncommon and often unavoidable if meticulous technique, appropriate preoperative planning, and close post-operative care are used. The keys to successfully managing complications that arise are having a thorough understanding of their cause and a defined treatment algorithm to obtain the best outcome.

REFERENCES

1. Gasques JA, Pereira de Godoy JM, Cruz EM. Psychosocial effects of otoplasty in children with prominent ears. Aesthetic Plast Surg 2008;32(6): 910–4.
2. Hauben DJ. Sushruta Samhita (Sushruta'a Collection) (800-600 B.C.?). Pioneers of plastic surgery. Acta Chir Plast 1984;26(2):65–8.
3. Goldwyn RM. Johann Friedrich Dieffenbach (1794-1847). Plast Reconstr Surg 1968;42(1):19–28.
4. Papel ID, editor. Facial plastic and reconstructive surgery. 3rd edition. New York: Thieme; 2009.
5. Janz BA, Cole P, Hollier LH Jr, et al. Treatment of prominent and constricted ear anomalies. Plast Reconstr Surg 2009;124(Suppl 1):27e–37e.
6. Nazarian R, Eshraghi AA. Otoplasty for the protruded ear. Semin Plast Surg 2011;25(4):288–94.
7. Furnas DW. Correction of prominent ears with multiple sutures. Clin Plast Surg 1978;5(3):491–5.
8. Mustarde JC. The correction of prominent ears using simple mattress sutures. Br J Plast Surg 1963;16: 170–8.
9. Adamson PA, Litner JA. Otoplasty technique. Facial Plast Surg Clin North Am 2006;14(2):79–87, v.
10. Limandjaja GC, Breugem CC, Mink van der Molen AB, et al. Complications of otoplasty: a literature review. J Plast Reconstr Aesthet Surg 2009; 62(1):19–27.
11. Owsley TG, Biggerstaff TG. Otoplasty complications. Oral Maxillofac Surg Clin North Am 2009; 21(1):105–18, vii.
12. Berghaus A, Braun T, Hempel JM. Revision otoplasty: how to manage the disastrous result. Arch Facial Plast Surg 2012;14(3):205–10.
13. Goode RL, Proffitt SD, Rafaty FM. Complications of otoplasty. Arch Otolaryngol 1970;91(4):352–5.
14. Goldwyn RM, Cohen MN. The unfavorable result in plastic surgery: avoidance and treatment. 3rd edition. Lippincott Williams & Wilkins; 2001.
15. Lentz AK, Plikaitis CM, Bauer BS. Understanding the unfavorable result after otoplasty: an integrated approach to correction. Plast Reconstr Surg 2011; 128(2):536–44.
16. Adamson PA, Strecker HD. Otoplasty techniques. Facial Plast Surg 1995;11(4):284–300.
17. Meyers EM, editor. Operative otolaryngology: head and neck surgery: expert consult: online, print and video, 2-volume set, 2e. 2nd edition. Philadelphia: Saunders; 2008.

Complications from Toxins and Fillers in the Dermatology Clinic
Recognition, Prevention, and Treatment

Steven H. Dayan, MD[a,b,c],*

KEYWORDS

- Cosmetic surgery complications • Toxin complications • Filler complications
- Cosmetic surgery safety

KEY POINTS

- Although counterfeit neurotoxin is available through Internet resources, it may not contain the amount of toxin stated on the label; risk of hurting patients makes the use of these products highly unethical.
- Adverse events with cosmetic use of neurotoxins and with fillers are commonly associated with intramuscular injections: local pain, infection, inflammation, tenderness, edema, erythema, bleeding, and ecchymosis.

INTRODUCTION
Toxins

Background

Forms of botulinum toxin type A (BoNTA) available for cosmetic use include onabotulinumtoxinA (Botox Cosmetic, Allergan, Irvine, CA), abobotulinumtoxinA (Dysport, Medicis Aesthetics, Scottsdale, AZ) and incobotulinumtoxinA (Xeomin, Merz Pharmaceuticals, Greensboro, NC). All of them are produced from fermentation of *Clostridium botulinum* type A (Hall strain) and may[1,2] or may not[3] contain accessory or hemagglutinin proteins. Other products marketed for medical (non-cosmetic) purposes include onabotulinumtoxinA (Botox) and rimabotulinumtoxinB (Myobloc), which is produced by fermentation of the bacterium *Clostridium botulinum* type B (Bean strain). Units of potency are specific to each BoNTA product, and the doses or units of biological activity cannot be compared or converted from 1 product to another.

It is important to use only BoNTA products that are approved by the US Food and Drug Administration (FDA). Counterfeit neurotoxin is available through Internet resources and may not contain the amount of toxin stated on the label.[4] Although these products can be bought at a reduced price, the risk of hurting patients makes the use of these products highly unethical.

Pharmacology

All BoNTA molecules consist of 1 heavy chain and 1 light chain polypeptide linked by a disulfide bond. They all share the same 3-step mechanism of action, which inhibits release of acetylcholine from peripheral cholinergic nerve endings at the neuromuscular junction.[5] First, the heavy chain binds to specific surface receptors on nerve endings. The BoNTA molecule then undergoes internalization via receptor-mediated endocytosis and the disulfide bond is cleaved. The light chain undergoes translocation to the cytosol, where it

[a] Chicago Center for Facial Plastic Surgery, Chicago, IL, USA; [b] DeNova Research, Chicago, IL, USA; [c] Department of Otolaryngology, University of Illinois at Chicago, Chicago, IL, USA
* Water Tower Place, 845 North Michigan Avenue, Suite 923, Chicago, IL 60611.
E-mail address: SDayan@DrDayan.com

Facial Plast Surg Clin N Am 21 (2013) 663–673
http://dx.doi.org/10.1016/j.fsc.2013.07.008
1064-7406/13/$ – see front matter © 2013 Elsevier Inc. All rights reserved.

cleaves polypeptides essential for docking, fusion, and release of acetylcholine vesicles through the cell membrane, resulting in chemical denervation of the muscle. Recovery of neurotransmission occurs as the neuromuscular junction recovers from SNAP25 cleavage and as new nerve endings are formed.

Postmarketing safety

Despite the potent systemic toxicity of BoNTA, the intramuscular injection of cosmetic BoNTA has an acceptable safety profile, with one of the largest known therapeutic indices for a prescription drug. It is one of the most studied pharmaceutical agents, with more than 3000 peer-reviewed published articles and more than 30 years of clinical experience. More than 10 million BoNTA treatments were performed worldwide last year. When used according to appropriate standards of care, it is the opinion of this author that BoNTA is one of the safest pharmaceutical agents available. Adverse events related to the cosmetic use of BoNTA reported to the FDA over a 13.5-year period included 36 serious and 995 nonserious adverse events.[6] There were no reported deaths. The nonserious adverse events consisted mainly of lack of effect (N = 623; 63%) and injection site reaction (N = 190; 19%).

In contrast, there were 406 reported adverse events related to the use of BoNTA for therapeutic or medical uses, such as cervical dystonia and cerebral palsy. These adverse events included 217 serious adverse events, including 28 deaths caused by respiratory, myocardial infarction, cerebrovascular accident, pulmonary embolism, and pneumonia[6]; however, many of these patients already had underlying disease, which likely led to or precipitated these serious events. The serious adverse events associated with medical uses of BoNTA are often caused by the use of higher doses used to treat large muscles and diffusion or the spread of the toxin away from the injection site[7] or the result of systemic toxicity.[8] Among patients treated for spasticity with BoNTA, the mean dose of onabotulinumtoxinA was 245 units (standard deviation [SD] 118 units) and abobotulinumtoxinA was 939 units (SD 324 units).[9] In contrast, it is uncommon to use more than 50 units cosmetically.

As a result of these reports, the FDA introduced several revisions to the prescribing information of BoNTA products (including aesthetic products), which includes a Boxed Warning highlighting the possibility of potentially life-threatening effects of distant spread of toxin after local injection, a Risk Evaluation and Mitigation Strategy, which includes a Medication Guide to help patients understand the risks and benefits of botulinum toxin products,

and changes to the established drug names to reinforce individual potencies and prevent medication errors.[10]

Indications

With respect to cosmetic use, BoNTA is indicated for the temporary improvement in the appearance of moderate to severe glabellar lines associated with corrugator or procerus muscle activity in adult patients aged 65 years or older[1-3]; however, off-label use is widespread and includes the treatment of forehead lines, crow's feet, bunny lines, upper and lower perioral lip lines, gingival smile, marionette lines, dimpled chin, and vertical neck lines.[11] Its effectiveness and safety in patients older than 65 years has also been shown.

Contraindications

The use of BoNTA is contraindicated in patients with an infection at the proposed site of injection and in individuals with known hypersensitivity to any botulinum toxin preparation[1-3] or to any of the components in the formulation, including albumin[1,3] and cow's milk protein,[2] because serious allergic reactions may occur. Although BoNTA is not recommended for use during pregnancy,[1-3] there are reports of BoNTA administration during pregnancy for medical conditions without apparent complications.[12] It is unknown whether BoNTA is excreted in breast milk.

Precautions

Because BoNTA diminishes neurotransmitter signaling at the neuromuscular junction, it should be used cautiously in patients with preexisting neuromuscular diseases, such as amyotrophic lateral sclerosis, myasthenia gravis, or Lambert-Eaton myasthenic syndrome.[1-3,5] The use of BoNTA has unmasked subclinical Lambert-Eaton myasthenic syndrome.[13] Similarly, patients may experience exaggerated effects in the presence of neuromuscular junction blockers, such as succinylcholine chloride, or other drugs that may interfere with neuromuscular transmission, including aminoglycosides, polymyxin, cyclosporin, chloroquine, quinidine, magnesium sulfate, and acetylcholinesterases.[1-3,5] The use of anticholinergic drugs after BoNTA administration may potentiate their systemic anticholinergic effects.[2,3]

Common adverse events

Common adverse events include local pain, infection, inflammation, tenderness, edema, erythema, bleeding, and ecchymosis, which are commonly associated with intramuscular injections. Other potential concerns include pain and infection.[14] Bruising is of particular concern in the crow's feet/lateral canthus/orbicularis oculi region.

Ecchymosis occurs most frequently in this region, because of the delicate and highly vascular nature of this tissue.[15] During clinical studies, bruising and pain were reported to occur in 6% to 25% of treated patients.[16,17]

Reports of temporary hypoesthesia at the injection site may be related to local needle trauma and edema but does not seem to be caused by nerve injury.[18] Uncommon psoriasiform eruptions[19] and skin dryness and flakiness[20] in the treated area may be caused by changes in skin secretions caused by BoNTA.[21] A potentially serious adverse event after BoNTA injection is severe headaches. Although not recognized in my own experience, 1 report[22] states that approximately 1% of treated patients developed headaches described as severe and debilitating. They spontaneously resolved after 2 to 4 weeks.

Unintended pharmacologic (toxic) effects

Although cosmetic BoNTA has an exceptional safety profile, misplaced injections may cause unwanted effects in nontarget areas. These effects may be the result of poor injection technique and failure to understand underlying facial anatomy. In addition to improper placement, unintended effects may also result from diffusion or spread of injected BoNTA into nearby functionally important muscle fibers. Injecting larger volumes of BoNTA results in greater diffusion, affecting a larger area.[23] The spread of toxin can also be affected by muscle contraction in the injected area.

Eyelid ptosis is a common complication of BoNTA injections and is most likely to be associated with injections of the orbicularis oculii, corrugator supercilii, and procerus muscles.[21] Eyelid ptosis may also result from BoNTA diffusion to the levator palpebrae superioris and may become apparent within 2 to 10 days of treatment and last approximately 2 to 4 weeks.[15] During 1 clinical trial,[24] blepharoptosis was reported to occur with a frequency of 5.4%. Overaggressive treatment of the frontalis muscles may also result in upper eyelid ptosis as well as brow ptosis.[15] Eyelid ptosis may be mistaken for myasthenia gravis.[25] It has been my impression that most incidences of eyelid ptosis after BoNTA injection are caused by unmasking underlying ptosis, which becomes more apparent after the reduction in muscle tone of the forehead together with the reduce compensatory lifting of the brow and upper eyelid. After the frontalis is weakened, preexisting ptosis becomes more obvious.

The injection of BoNTA in the lower eyelid area may adversely affect the function of the orbicularis oculi muscle. Although uncommon and unrecognized in more than 30,000 injections by me,

lagophthalmos after aesthetic procedures is reported to result from paralysis of the orbicularis oculi muscles, which decreases blink strength, and tonic orbicularis contraction, causing dry eyes. The resulting corneal exposure may cause superficial punctate keratitis.[26] Dry eyes in theory can also result from ectropion or abnormal eversion of the lower eyelid so that the inner surface is exposed[27]; however, a significant amount of neurotoxin would need to be injected periocularly and into the lower lid for this to occur. If it does occur, ectropion requires prompt medical attention to prevent exposure keratitis and corneal injury.

BoNTA injected into the periocular area can also adversely affect tear production, requiring the use of lubricating eye drops.[28] This situation is a result of obstruction of the tear canal caused by paralysis of the orbicularis muscle.[29] The effect of periocular BoNTA injection on tear production was studied in 13 women undergoing bilateral treatment of crow's feet.[30] The Schirmer test was used to assess tear production. Among the 26 treated eyes, 5 eyes of 3 patients had a significant decrease in Schirmer test results 1 month after injection and 3 eyes of 2 patients had a significant decrease in Schirmer test results at 4 months after injection; however, whether this is clinically significant is debatable, because only 1 patient reported dry-eye symptoms at 4 months.

Injection of BoNTA into the superior rectus muscle for the treatment of strabismus was one of the first therapeutic uses of botulinum toxins.[31] By injecting the toxin into the stronger muscle and weakening it, proper alignment of the eyes can be achieved. Temporary strabismus may also occur after BoNTA injections of the lateral canthal areas as a result of diffusion, causing weakness of the lateral rectus muscles.[21]

Upper lip ptosis has rarely been reported after the injection of BoNTA into the lateral canthal creases and orbicularis oculi muscle and may be related to prior blepharoplasty.[32] In these cases, evidence of lip weakness began after 7 to 10 days and resolved after 5 to 6 weeks. Lip weakness can also occur from perioral injections to soften radial perioral lines and lateral canthal areas. Correction of chin dimpling or peau d'orange skin can be achieved by injecting BoNTA into the medial mentalis muscle; however, lateral injection placement may affect the depressor labii muscles and result in lower lip ptosis.

Large doses of BoNTA injected into the platysma for the treatment of platysmal bands and horizontal neck lines can produce weakness of the neck flexors and dysphagia and hoarseness[27]; however, routine administration of 30 to 40 units has not resulted in adverse events.

Antibody formation

Formation of antibodies to abobotulinumtoxinA and onabotulinumtoxinA after cosmetic applications has occurred in only a few case reports[33] and seems to be more common with medical applications.[34] Although not a danger to the patient, the development of neutralizing antibodies in theory may limit the therapeutic effectiveness of BoNTA injections. In 1 report,[33] therapeutic failure caused by the development of BoNTA antibodies occurred in 4 patients after 3 to 13 injection sessions over 18 to 65 months, whereas a large meta-analysis[35] reported that 11 of 2240 treated patients (0.49%) became positive for onabotulinumtoxinA antibodies, but only 3 patients became clinically unresponsive to onabotulinumtoxinA.

Ultraviolet light exposure

Using the time course of anhydrosis after intradermal injection of BoNTA, excessive exposure to UV-B radiation reduced the area of sweating by approximately 30%, although the duration of effect remained unchanged.[36] These investigators suggested that exposure to UV-B radiation may result in denaturation or degradation of BoNTA.

Preventing common adverse events

To minimize the risk of bleeding and bruising, medications that may increase bleeding such as aspirin and nonsteroidal antiinflammatory drugs should be stopped at least 10 days before receiving BoNTA injections.[37] If a blood vessel is inadvertently punctured, applying immediate pressure on the injection site may help minimize the development of widespread ecchymosis.[21]

Injection discomfort may be reduced by the use of small-diameter needles, such as 30-gauge to 34-gauge,[37] and changing the needle after 3 or 4 injections.[21] It has been suggested[27] that pinching the skin and the underlying muscle to be injected and slowly injecting the BoNTA solution may help reduce injection pain. Using a similar technique was reported to significantly reduce pain and eliminate unpleasant crunchy sensations.[38]

The application of ice packs on the intended treatment area may also help minimize pain.[37] In 1 study,[39] the application of ice packs 5 minutes before periocular BoNTA injection decreased pain scores by 45%. In another study,[40] the application of ice packs 5 minutes before injecting the lateral canthus with BoNTA significantly diminished pain; however, others have reported that cooling provides only minimal pain relief from periocular BoNTA injections.[41] Topical application of an anesthetic cream has also been suggested to decrease injection pain.[27] The topical application of lidocaine 4% cream significantly reduced the pain associated with the injection of BoNTA in the lateral canthal areas.[42]

It has been suggested that differences in the diluents used to reconstitute BoNTA products may affect injection pain. The results of 2 studies[43,44] showed that reconstitution of BoNTA using a preservative-containing saline solution significantly decreased the perception of pain perception during multiple BoNTA injections.

Prevention of complications

It has been anecdotally reported that applying digital pressure between the injection site and the eye may reduce the spread of BoNTA. When injecting the glabellar area, the spread of BoNTA may be reduced by squeezing the corrugator muscle between 2 fingers while injecting, although this has not been proved, to my knowledge. Placing corrugator injections 1 cm or more above the supraorbital ridge and using smaller injection volumes also reduces the spread of BoNTA and minimizes the occurrence of eyelid ptosis.[21] The benefit of remaining upright for several hours after treatment remains unclear and likely has no effect on the toxin spread.

Patients with preexisting lower lid laxity such as the elderly may be at greater risk for ectropion. Before periorbital injections are administered, the snap test or lower lid extraction test may help identify patients at risk.[21] Periorbital complications can also be minimized by injecting outside the infraorbital rim or beyond 1 cm lateral to the lateral canthus. Strabismus and diplopia are unlikely during cosmetic injections and are caused by unwanted lateral rectus weakness; these conditions can be guarded against by avoiding injections within the orbital rim and perhaps by applying digital pressure to isolate the drug while injecting. Patients experiencing strabismus or diplopia may require an ophthalmology consultation.[21]

Lip dysfunction may be avoided by minimizing the number of perioral injections and keeping BoNTA injections 5 mm apart.[21] Noticeable brow ptosis can be avoided by conservatively treating the medial forehead and foregoing treatment of the lateral forehead in those with low brows; however, patients with lateral frontalis muscle hyperactivity may develop brow arching, which results in a joker face. These patients may require a dose of 1 to 2 U of onabotulinumtoxinA or 3 to 6 U of abobotulinumtoxinA just over the lateral brow. Close examination before treatment should identify at-risk patients.

Dermal Fillers

Background

The most commonly used dermal fillers are made of hyaluronic acid, a glycosaminoglycan consisting of repeating units of glucuronic acid and N-acetyl-glucosamine. When combined with water, hyaluronic acid forms a viscous gel. Because normal human skin consists to a large extent of hyaluronic acid, it is well suited for use in dermal fillers. Several hyaluronic acid–containing dermal fillers are commercially available (Restylane and Perlane, Medicis Aesthetics, Scottsdale, AZ; Juvéderm Ultra Plus, and Juvéderm Voluma, Allergan, Irvine, CA). These fillers are chemically similar but differ in their physical properties because of different manufacturing processes.[45] Hyaluronic acid dermal fillers may also contain lidocaine (Belotero and Belotero Balance; Merz Aesthetics and Juvéderm Ultra XC; Medicis Aesthetics, Scottsdale, AZ). Hyaluronic acid–containing dermal fillers are not permanent, because they undergo slow degradation by endogenous hyaluronidase.[46]

Calcium hydroxylapatite (Radiesse, Merz Aesthetics) is a suspension of 20-μM to 45-μM particles in a methylcellulose gel. When used for augmentation, it lasts for 10 to 14 months, but its duration has been reported to range significantly longer and shorter than this.[47] Poly-L-lactic acid (Sculptra Aesthetic, Sanofi-Aventis US) is a synthetic peptide polymer with particles sizes of 40 to 60 μM. Both calcium hydroxylapatite and poly-L-lactic acid stimulate collagen neogenesis[47] and are considered semipermanent. One product containing nonresorbable polymethylmethacrylate microspheres suspended in bovine collagen (Artefill, Suneva Medical) is considered a permanent facial filler. It also contains lidocaine.

Contraindications

Contraindications to the use of dermal fillers include hypersensitivity to product components, bleeding disorders, especially with use of cannulas, and a history of anaphylaxis or presence of multiple severe allergies. Because hyaluronic acid–containing products are made by bacterial fermentation, a history of allergy to gram-positive bacterial proteins has been suggested to be a contraindication to their use; however, this seems to be hypothetical. Polymethylmethacrylate is contraindicated for use in lip augmentation and injection into the vermilion or the wet mucosa of the lip.[48] Polymethylmethacrylate and poly-L-lactic acid should not be used in patients with known history of or susceptibility to keloid formation or hypertrophic scarring.[48,49]

Common adverse events

Similar to treatment with toxins, the introduction of needles into tissue may be associated with local pain, erythema, edema, and ecchymosis.[50–52]

Patients should be cautioned that that these responses may occur but are generally short-lived[53]; however, these can be reduced or eliminated by a proper injection technique.

I have avoided much of the discomfort associated with dermal filler injection by adopting the use of blunt-tip cannulas (SoftFil, AlphaMedix, Petah Tikva, Israel) for all areas of the face. These cannulas permit deeper placement of fillers, resulting in more immediate results, and virtually eliminate discomfort, bruising, and swelling. The cannula I prefer using is 22-gauge and 70 mm long. As the cannula advances through the facial plane, it gently pushes underlying soft tissue out of the way. By thinning products[54–56] with 1% lidocaine (0.3 mL), it becomes more malleable and it can be massaged into place after deep injection.

The decision whether to use an anesthetic depends on the patient, the product, and the area to be treated. Some products are manufactured with 0.3% dry preservative-free lidocaine,[54,55] which significantly reduces injection-related discomfort[57]; however, in my practice, I premix all filler products with 1% lidocaine. In addition to achieving an anesthetic effect, the addition of lidocaine decreases filler viscosity, further alleviating discomfort. By using blunt-tip cannulas, there is little discomfort when treating cheeks and tear trough, making anesthetics unnecessary.

For very pain-sensitive patients, I use a regional nerve block when treating the lower one-third of the face and especially the lips. I start by applying 2% benzocaine paste (Hurricane, Beutlich Pharmaceuticals, Waukegan, IL) with a cotton swab along the oral buccal mucosal. Five minutes later, I apply 4 intraoral injections of mepivicaine HCl 3% (Isocaine, Henry Schein, Melville, NY) (2 superior and 2 inferior), anesthetizing the labial branches of the inferior orbital nerve and the mental nerves. Mepivicaine is short acting (~30 minutes) and better tolerated than lidocaine.

A useful technique for avoiding pain is applying a vibrating nerve distracter near and above the injection point during anesthetic injection. Patients are often are unaware that they have been injected. For patients who are resistant to nerve blocks, I apply topical 30% lidocaine cream (SCP, Sherman Oaks, CA) for 20 to 30 minutes. This technique is especially effective for use on the lips, where I place the cream into a special mouth guard, which keeps the product over the labial mucosa.

Complications

Although occurring with an incidence of only 0.001%,[58] focal necrosis has been associated with dermal fillers of all types[59] and represents a serious complication. The vascular nature of the glabella makes it the most common site of necrosis caused by intra-arterial injection of dermal fillers,[60] but intra-arterial injection in the nasolabial fold has also been reported.[61,62] Inadvertent intra-arterial injection of a polymethylmethacrylate dermal filler in the glabellar area for soft tissue augmentation resulted in blindness and total ophthalmoplegia.[63] These investigators speculated that the injected material entered a peripheral branch of the ophthalmic artery or some anastomosing artery, from where it traveled to the ophthalmic artery and reached the retinal central artery and anterior and long posterior ciliary arteries, where it resulted in blindness, corneal and iris ischemia, and total ophthalmoplegia.

In my experience, the appearance of impending tissue necrosis occurs immediately, within 24 to 48 hours, or is delayed. Occlusion caused by direct intravascular injection results in immediate blanching. Although aspirating before injecting may help prevent intravascular injection, it is difficult to perform with the current filler products. I find it helpful to inject slowly (less than 0.3 mL/min), keep the needle in motion, and avoid injecting near large facial vessels. As mentioned earlier, I premix filler products with 0.3 mL of lidocaine before injection to decrease its viscosity and minimize the risk for occlusion; however, the likely cause of reported necrosis is tissue pressure secondary to local edema or the hydrophilic properties of the product-occluding vessels. For this reason, the onset of symptoms may be delayed 24 to 48 hours.

I have modified a previously published protocol[64] for the recognition and treatment of impending necrosis from soft tissue filler injection with satisfactory results (**Table 1**). Blanching followed by a dusky or purple discoloration of the injected area indicates vascular compromise.[65] Regardless of filler type, the injection should be immediately stopped and 10 to 30 units of hyaluronidase diluted 1:1 with saline should be injected into each 2-cm × 2-cm area of affected tissue. Because hypersensitivity reactions can occur, skin should be tested before hyaluronidase is injected.[65,66] Hyaluronidase is also effective for reducing rejection-induced edema.[67] It is likely that an inflammatory response causes an increase in hyaluronan via cytokines and growth factor, which is then mitigated by the hyaluronidase.[68] It is for this reason that I believe it to be effective for the treatment of impending necrosis caused by all filler products, regardless of type.

The application of 2% nitroglycerin paste (Nitro-BID, E. Fougera, Melville, NY) to the area of impending necrosis may also be beneficial. The product should be applied daily to the affected area until the capillary refill rate exceeds 2 seconds; however, the use of large amounts of 2% nitroglycerin paste (>1.25 cm [0.5 inch]) may cause systemic effects. Warm compresses may also provide vasodilatation, and daily aspirin may prevent further clot formation. Patients are followed daily for further signs of occlusion or necrosis. If edema is slow to resolve, methylprednisolone is added. Hyperbaric oxygen should be considered if the affected area does not respond to these treatments (**Fig. 1**).

At one time, the reported rate of hypersensitivity reactions to hyaluronic acid was 0.07%, but it has decreased to 0.02%, because more highly purified products contain lower amounts of protein.[69] Immediate hypersensitivity reactions are rarely

Table 1	
Recognition and treatment of impending necrosis	
Presentation	Immediate or early blanching followed by a dusky or purple discoloration of the area
Treatment	Discontinue injection Perform hyaluronidase skin testing Inject 10–30 U of hyaluronidase per 2-cm² area Massage 1.25 cm (0.5 inch) of 2% nitroglycerin paste into the area and apply warm compresses Begin aspirin 325 mg and an antacid regimen Apply topical oxygen cosmeceutical therapy twice daily
Additional management	Follow patient daily for further signs of occlusion/necrosis Continue hyaluronidase and 2% nitroglycerin paste daily as needed Continue aspirin, antacid, and topical oxygen therapy until wound has healed If edema progresses, place on tapering doses of methylprednisolone Consider hyperbaric oxygen for progressing necrosis resistant to above treatments

From Dayan SH, Arkins JP, Mathison CC. Management of impending necrosis associated with soft tissue filler injections. J Drugs Dermatol 2011;10:1007–12; with permission.

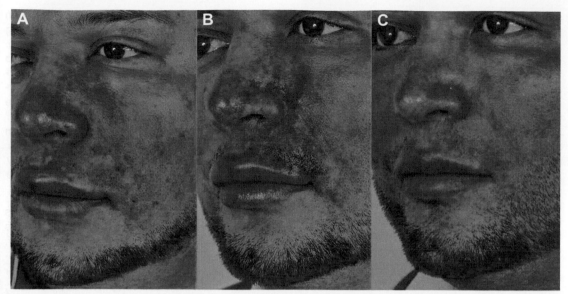

Fig. 1. (*A*) Vascular reticulated pattern commonly seen within 24 hours after intravascular injection of filler. It is important to recognize this subtle but critical sign, which may indicate a serious vascular occlusion. (*B*) Forty-eight hours after injections after institution of impending necrosis treatments as per protocol (see **Table 1**), extensive necrosis is averted. (*C*) Routine follow-up 5 months later with no evidence of injury.

severe[51] and are more likely to occur with bovine-derived products. Immediate hypersensitivity reactions are also more common with products containing a local anesthetic.[51] Reports of angioedema are rare.[70]

Many reactions that are assumed to be allergic or hypersensitivity responses are most likely caused by bacterial reactions.[71] Local infections are rare but have been associated with the use of unapproved products.[72] Biofilms can present as

Table 2	
Prevention and treatment of hypersensitivity reactions/infections	
Before treatment	Cleanse the face thoroughly of all makeup before injection
	Use benzalkonium chloride wash or povidone-iodine (Betadine) swab to prepare the face just before the treatment
	Use as few injection sites as possible
	Avoid bolus injections
	Avoid injecting into previously placed fillers or through infected tissue
	Avoid injecting through oral or nasal mucosa
	Consider prophylactic antibiotics before a dental procedure or if a facial infection occurs within 2 wk of a filler treatment
If a red indurated area appears any time after the treatment, regardless of duration	Inject hyaluronidase regardless of filler used 10–30 units mixed 1:1 with saline (Vitrase, ISTA Pharmaceuticals, Irvine, CA)
	Start antibiotics: ciprofloxacin 500 mg QD (Cipro, Bayer HealthCare Pharmaceuticals, Wayne, NJ) and clarithromycin 500 mg twice daily (Biaxin, Abbott Laboratories, Abbott Park, IL)
	Avoid all forms of steroids or nonsteroidal antiinflammatory drugs
If long-term indurated area or steroids have already been used	Inject 15–40 mg fluorouracil (APP Pharmaceuticals, Schaumburg, IL)
	Repeat every 4 wk
If induration remains persistent despite fluorouracil treatment	Consider laser lysis
	Consider incision and washing out cavity with antibiotics
	Surgical excision as last resort

sterile abscesses or chronic inflammation and infections[73] and may cause a foreign body response, resembling an allergic reaction.[74,75] Treatment of early infectious complications from biofilm reactions included broad-spectrum antibiotics such as fluoroquinolone or macrolide antibiotics.[76]

In 1 case report, poly-L-lactic acid was used to treat facial lipodystrophy associated with human immunodeficiency virus.[77] Approximately 1 year after the last treatment, the patient complained of hot, hard, painful, and distorting bumps at the injection sites. Examination of the patient revealed warm, erythematous, and fibrotic skin and nodules located on treated areas, which were attributed to a delayed allergic reaction. I believe that hypersensitivity reactions are likely to have an infectious cause and I have developed a protocol for the prevention and treatment of hypersensitivity/infectious reactions (**Table 2**).

Cosmetic complications

Light refraction through improperly injected dermal filler, especially hyaluronic acid–containing products, may cause bluish discoloration, known as the Tyndall effect. The risk of this discoloration can be prevented or minimized by avoiding superficial placement.[53,78] If undesirable placement occurs, the gel can be thinly distributed by massage or it can be removed with a needle or by excision.[53] Hyaluronic acid is highly hygroscopic, and depending on whether the hyaluronic acid filler is maximally hydrated, some swelling of the material may occur after injection. Depending on the injection site, this swelling may result in excessive fullness in areas of loose tissue, such as lower eyelids and lips. White nodules may be visible if particulate fillers are injected too superficially (**Fig. 2**).[64,78]

The use of excessive amounts of dermal fillers can result in poor cosmetic outcomes. For example, overfilling of the nasolabial folds can result in a simian appearance, whereas overfilling of lips leads to a shelflike sausage appearance. This highly unnatural look makes it apparent to others that a cosmetic procedure has been performed. Lumps may respond to massage[64] or hyaluronidase can be used to break down excessive or misplaced hyaluronic acid–containing fillers.[66] Other alternatives include aspiration or incision and drainage.[64]

SUMMARY

Although the use of BoNTA for cosmetic use has an outstanding safety profile, adverse reactions and unintended effects can occasionally occur. Patients requiring high doses and those with preexisting neuromuscular disorders are at greater risk of BoNTA-related complications; however, these can be minimized or eliminated by proper injection techniques and conservative dosing. As the use of fillers becomes increasingly more common, adverse events can be expected to increase as well; however, many complications can be avoided with appropriate training and proper injection techniques.

REFERENCES

1. Botox® [package insert]. Irvine (CA): Allergan Pharm; 2011.
2. Dysport® [package insert]. Scottsdale (AZ): Medicis Aesthetics; 2009.
3. Xeomin® [Package insert]. Franksville (WI): Merz Pharm; 2011.
4. Pickett A. Serious issues relating to counterfeit dermal fillers available from Internet sources. J Am Acad Dermatol 2009;65:642–3.
5. Huang W, Foster JA, Rogachefsky AS. Pharmacology of botulinum toxin. J Am Acad Dermatol 2000;43(2 Pt 1):249–59.
6. Coté TR, Mohan AK, Polder JA, et al. Botulinum toxin type A injections: adverse events reported to the US Food and Drug Administration in therapeutic and cosmetic cases. J Am Acad Dermatol 2005;53:407–15.
7. Coban A, Matur Z, Hanagasi HA, et al. Iatrogenic botulism after botulinum toxin type A injections. Clin Neuropharmacol 2010;33:158–60.
8. Crowner BE, Brunstrom JE, Racette BA. Iatrogenic botulism due to therapeutic botulinum toxin a injection in a pediatric patient. Clin Neuropharmacol 2007;30:310–3.
9. Roche N, Schnitzler A, Genêt FF, et al. Undesirable distant effects following botulinum toxin type a injection. Clin Neuropharmacol 2008;31:272–80.

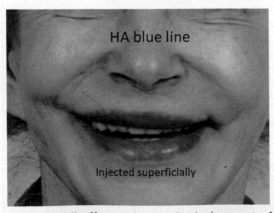

Fig. 2. Tyndall effect with superficial placement of hyaluronic filler.

10. Kuehn BM. FDA requires black box warnings on labeling for botulinum toxin products. JAMA 2009; 301:2316.

11. Kane M, Donofrio L, Ascher B, et al. Expanding the use of neurotoxins in facial aesthetics: a consensus panel's assessment and recommendations. J Drugs Dermatol 2010;9(Suppl):S7–22.

12. Morgan JC, Iyer SS, Moser ET, et al. Botulinum toxin A during pregnancy: a survey of treating physicians. J Neurol Neurosurg Psychiatry 2006;77: 117–9.

13. Erbguth F, Claus D, Engelhardt A, et al. Systemic effect of local botulinum toxin injections unmasks subclinical Lambert-Eaton myasthenic syndrome. J Neurol Neurosurg Psychiatry 1993;56:1235–6.

14. Dutton J, Fowler A. Botulinum toxin in ophthalmology. Surv Ophthalmol 2007;52:13–31.

15. Pena M, Alam M, Yoo S. Complications with the use of botulinum toxin type A for cosmetic applications and hyperhidrosis. Semin Cutan Med Surg 2007; 26:29–33.

16. Lowe N, Lask G, Yamauchi P, et al. Bilateral, double-blind, randomized comparison of 3 doses of botulinum toxin type A and placebo in patients with crow's feet. J Am Acad Dermatol 2002;47: 834–40.

17. Lowe N, Ascher B, Heckmann M, et al. Double-blind, randomized, placebo-controlled, dose-response study of the safety and officacy of botulinum toxin type A In subjects with crow's feet. Dermatol Surg 2005;31:257–62.

18. Lu L, Atchabahian A, Mackinnon SE, et al. Nerve injection injury with botulinum toxin. Plast Reconstr Surg 1998;101:1875–80.

19. Bowden JB, Rapini RP. Psoriasiform eruption from intramuscular botulinum A toxin. Cutis 1992;50: 415–6.

20. Bulstrode NW, Grobelaar AO. Long-term prospective follow-up of botulinum toxin treatment for facial rhytids. Aesthetic Plast Surg 2002;26:356–9.

21. Vartanian AJ, Dayan SH. Complications of botulinum toxin A use in facial rejuvenation. Facial Plast Surg Clin North Am 2005;13:1–10.

22. Alam M. Severe, intractable headache after injection with botulinum A exotoxin: report of 5 cases. J Am Acad Dermatol 2002;46:62–5.

23. Hsu TS, Dover JS, Arndt KA. Effect of volume and concentration on the diffusion of botulinum exotoxin A. Arch Dermatol 2004;140:1351–4.

24. Carruthers JA, Lowe NJ, Menter MA, et al. A multicenter, double-blind, randomized, placebo-controlled study of the efficacy and safety of botulinum toxin type A in the treatment of glabellar lines. J Am Acad Dermatol 2002;46:840–9.

25. Parikh R, Lavin PJ. Cosmetic botulinum toxin type A induced ptosis presenting as myasthenia. Ophthal Plast Reconstr Surg 2011;27:470.

26. Northington ME, Huang CC. Dry eyes and superficial punctate keratitis: a complication of treatment of glabelar dynamic rhytides with botulinum exotoxin A. Dermatol Surg 2004;30(Pt 2):1515–7.

27. Klein AW. Contraindications and complications with the use of botulinum toxin. Clin Dermatol 2004;22: 66–75.

28. Matarasso S. Decreased tear expression with an abnormal Schirmer's test following botulinum toxin type A for the treatment of lateral canthal rhytides. Dermatol Surg 2002;28:149–52.

29. Keegan DJ, Geerling G, Lee JP, et al. Botulinum toxin treatment for hyperlacrimation secondary to aberrant regenerated seventh nerve palsy or salivary gland transplantation. Br J Ophthalmol 2002; 86:43–6.

30. Arat Y, Yen M. Effect of botulinum toxin type A on tear production after treatment of lateral canthal rhytids. Ophthal Plast Reconstr Surg 2007;23:22–4.

31. Scott AB. Botulinum toxin injection of eye muscles to correct strabismus. Trans Am Ophthalmol Soc 1981;79:734–70.

32. Matarasso S, Matarasso A. Treatment guidelines for botulinum toxin type A for the periocular region and a report on partial upper lip ptosis following injections to the lateral canthal rhytids. Plast Reconstr Surg 2001;108:208–14.

33. Dressler D, Wohlfahrt K, Meyer-Rogge E, et al. Antibody-induced failure of botulinum toxin A therapy in cosmetic indications. Dermatol Surg 2010; 36(Suppl 4):2182–7.

34. Greene P, Fahn S, Diamond B. Development of resistance to botulinum toxin type A in patients with torticollis. Mov Disord 1994;9:213–7.

35. Naumann M, Carruthers A, Carruthers J, et al. Meta-analysis of neutralizing antibody conversion with onabotulinumtoxinA (BOTOX®) across multiple indications. Mov Disord 2010;25:2211–8.

36. Sycha T, Kotzailias N, Kranz G, et al. UV-B irradiation attenuates dermal effects of botulinum toxin A: a randomized, double-blind, placebo-controlled study. Dermatol Surg 2007;33(1 Spec No):S92–6.

37. Wollina U, Konrad H. Managing adverse events associated with botulinum toxin type A: a focus on cosmetic procedures. Am J Clin Dermatol 2005;6:141–50.

38. Seiger ES, Stephenson SR. Using manual tissue stabilization (the "no crunch" method) for reduction of pain in botulinum toxin injections. J Am Osteopath Dermatol 2007;8:64.

39. Linder JS, Edmonson BC, Laquis SJ, et al. Skin cooling before periocular botulinum toxin A injection. Ophthal Plast Reconstr Surg 2002;18: 441–2.

40. Sarifakioglu N, Sarifakioglu E. Evaluating the effects of ice application on the pain felt during botulinum toxin type-A injections: a prospective,

randomized, single-blind controlled trial. Ann Plast Surg 2004;53:543–6.

41. Beer KR, Wilson F. Skin cooling provides minimal relief of patient discomfort during periocular botulinum toxin type A injection. Dermatol Surg 2011;37:870–2.

42. Carruthers A, Carruthers J. Single-center, double-blind, randomized study to evaluate the efficacy of 4% lidocaine cream versus vehicle cream during botulinum toxin type A treatments. Dermatol Surg 2005;31:165–9.

43. Alam M, Dover JS, Arndt KA. Pain associated with injection of botulinum toxin A exotoxin reconstituted using isotonic sodium chloride with and without preservative. Arch Dermatol 2002;138:510–4.

44. Sarifakioglu N, Sarifakioglu E. Evaluating effects of preservative-containing saline solution on pain perception during botulinum toxin type-A injections at different locations: a prospective, single-blinded, randomized controlled trial. Aesthetic Plast Surg 2005;29:113–5.

45. Stocks D, Sundaram H, Michaels J, et al. Rheological evaluation of the physical properties of hyaluronic acid dermal fillers. J Drugs Dermatol 2011;10:974–80.

46. Tezel A, Fredrickson GH. The science of hyaluronic acid dermal fillers. J Cosmet Laser Ther 2008;10:35–42.

47. Bentkover SH. The biology of facial fillers. Facial Plast Surg 2009;25:73–85.

48. Artefill® [Package insert]. San Diego (CA): Suneva Medical; 2010.

49. Sculptra® Aesthetic [Package insert]. Bridgewater (NJ): Sanofi-Aventis US.

50. Andre P, Lowe NJ, Parc A, et al. Adverse reactions to dermal fillers: a review of European experiences. J Cosmet Laser Ther 2005;7:171–6.

51. Lowe NJ, Maxwell CA, Patnaik R. Adverse reactions to dermal fillers: review. Dermatol Surg 2005;31(11 Pt 2):1616–25.

52. Glogau RG, Kane MA. Effect of injection techniques on the rate of local adverse events in patients implanted with nonanimal hyaluronic acid gel dermal fillers. Dermatol Surg 2008;34(Suppl 1):S105–9.

53. Bailey SH, Cohen JL, Kenkel JM. Etiology, prevention, and treatment of dermal filler complications. Aesthet Surg J 2011;31:110–21.

54. Juvéderm® Ultra XC [Package insert]. Irvine (CA): Allergan Pharm.

55. Restylane® [Package insert]. Scottsdale (AZ): Medicis Aesthetics; 2011.

56. Radiesse® [Package insert]. San Mateo (CA): Merz Aesthetics.

57. Weinkle SH, Bank DE, Boyd CM, et al. A multi-center, double-blind, randomized controlled study of the safety and effectiveness of Juvederm injectable gel with and without lidocaine. J Cosmet Dermatol 2009;8(3):205–10.

58. Hanke CW, Higley HR, Jolivette DM, et al. Abscess formation and local necrosis after treatment with Zyderm or Zyplast collagen implant. J Am Acad Dermatol 1991;25(2 Pt 1):319–26.

59. Narins RS, Jewell M, Rubin M, et al. Clinical conference: management of rare events following dermal fillers–focal necrosis and angry red bumps. Dermatol Surg 2006;32:426–34.

60. Glaich AS, Cohen JL, Goldberg LH. Injection necrosis of the glabella: protocol for prevention and treatment after use of dermal fillers. Dermatol Surg 2006;32:276–81.

61. Dayan SH, Arkins JP, Mathison CC. Management of impending necrosis associated with soft tissue filler injections. J Drugs Dermatol 2011;10:1007–12.

62. Kang MS, Park ES, Shin HS, et al. Skin necrosis of the nasal ala after injection of dermal fillers. Dermatol Surg 2011;37:375–80.

63. Silva MT, Curi AL. Blindness and total ophthalmoplegia after aesthetic polymethylmethacrylate injection: case report. Arq Neuropsiquiatr 2004;62:873–4.

64. Cohen JL. Understanding, avoiding, and managing dermal filler complications. Dermatol Surg 2008;34(Suppl 1):S92–9.

65. Grunebaum LD, Bogdan Allemann I, Dayan S, et al. The risk of alar necrosis associated with dermal filler injection. Dermatol Surg 2009;35(Suppl 2):1635–40.

66. Brody HJ. Use of hyaluronidase in the treatment of granulomatous hyaluronic acid reactions or unwanted hyaluronic acid misplacement. Dermatol Surg 2005;31:893–7.

67. Johnsson C, Hallgren R, Elvin A, et al. Hyaluronidase ameliorates rejection-induced edema. Transpl Int 1999;12:235–43.

68. Engstrom-Laurent A, Feltelius N, Hallgren R, et al. Raised serum hyaluronate levels in scleroderma: an effect of growth factor induced activation of connective tissue cells? Ann Rheum Dis 1985;44:614–20.

69. Friedman PM, Mafong EA, Kauvar AN, et al. Safety data of injectable nonanimal stabilized hyaluronic acid gel for soft tissue augmentation. Dermatol Surg 2002;28:491–4.

70. Leonhardt JM, Lawrence N, Narins RS. Angioedema acute hypersensitivity reaction to injectable hyaluronic acid. Dermatol Surg 2005;31:577–9.

71. Dayan SH, Arkins JP, Brindise R. Soft tissue fillers and biofilms. Facial Plast Surg 2011;27:23–8.

72. Toy BR, Frank PJ. Outbreak of Mycobacterium abscessus infection after soft tissue augmentation. Dermatol Surg 2003;29:971–3.

73. Dijkema SJ, van der Lei B, Kibbelaar RE. New-fill injections may induce late-onset foreign body granulomatous reaction. Plast Reconstr Surg 2005;115:76e–8e.

74. Christensen L, Breiting V, Janssen M, et al. Adverse reactions to injectable soft tissue permanent fillers. Aesthetic Plast Surg 2005;29:34–48.

75. Christensen L. Normal and pathologic tissue reactions to soft tissue gel fillers. Dermatol Surg 2007; 33(Suppl 2):S168–75.

76. Bjarnsholt T, Tolker-Nielsen T, Givskov M, et al. Detection of bacteria by fluorescence in situ hybridization in culture-negative soft tissue filler lesions. Dermatol Surg 2009;35(Suppl 2):1620–4.

77. Dayan SH, Antonucci CM, Stephany M. Painful red, hot bumps after injectable poly-L-lactic acid treatment: a case report. Cosmet Derm 2008;21:388–90.

78. Sclafani AP, Fagien S. Treatment of injectable soft tissue filler complications. Dermatol Surg 2009; 35(Suppl 2):1672–80.

Complications in Hair Restoration

Samuel M. Lam, MD

KEYWORDS

- Cosmetic complications • Hair transplant • Hair restoration • Plugs • Pitting • Cobblestoning
- Compression • Hairline

KEY POINTS

- A surgeon must treat the donor area with commensurate respect to the recipient area and carefully harvest hair so as to avoid transection of hair, transection of nerve and blood supply, and tension.
- The surgeon must learn how to create hairlines that are natural macroscopically (position, tilt, shape) and microscopically (angle, distribution, mimicking a coastline).
- The surgeon must understand how to create recipient sites that are angled and directed to follow the natural flow of hairs on a head.
- Assistants must practice meticulous graft dissection and placement so as to generate grafts that are minimally manipulated and that are placed into the correct site with the right fit, direction, and so on.

INTRODUCTION

Too often many facial plastic surgeons who are highly skilled in their craft endeavor to enter the world of hair restoration without proper training or understanding, which can lead to a myriad of untoward complications. Unfortunately, hair restoration has been viewed with a haughtiness that it is an inferior surgical discipline as compared with, for instance, the delicate task of rhinoplasty and, with that hubris, one can unwittingly stray into problems, some of which may not even be recognized as a complication because of an inability to recognize it as such. In this article, common types of complications in hair transplant surgery, divided into those of the donor site versus the recipient site, are reviewed. Common causes, how to avoid such complications, as well as possible solutions once they have occurred are also reviewed.

SURGICAL COMPLICATIONS
Donor Site

Complications

- Poor wound healing/scarring (atrophic, widened, hypertrophic, hypopigmented)
- Necrosis
- Chronic pain

Cause Improper donor harvesting (too wide a scar, too much tension, poor location, transection of hair follicles, transection of blood and nerve supply, improper undermining).

Avoidance Surgical complications can be avoided by paying attention to the depth and angle of one's harvest (staying within the subcutaneous plane and above the galea), avoiding transection of the underlying blood supply, nerves, galea,

Disclosures: None.
Lam Institute for Hair Restoration, 6101 Chapel Hill Boulevard, Suite 101, Plano, TX 75093, USA
E-mail address: drlam@lamfacialplastics.com

Facial Plast Surg Clin N Am 21 (2013) 675–680
http://dx.doi.org/10.1016/j.fsc.2013.07.010
1064-7406/13/$ – see front matter © 2013 Elsevier Inc. All rights reserved.

and surrounding hairs. It should be ascertained there is sufficient laxity (preoperative scalp relaxation exercises in a tense scalp), sufficient time between operative harvesting cases so that the scalp has had time to relax, and only 1 cm or less in width should be harvested when removing a donor strip. Use of tumescent solution to help straighten follicles and to limit injury to the underlying nerve and blood supply is critical. A careful 2-layered closure is helpful to minimize scarring. Use of platelet-rich plasma (PRP) can help with good wound healing. If a wound is under tension, the wound should be closed in a delayed fashion rather than undermined or forcefully drawn close, both of which can lead to necrosis, unpredictable hair loss in the donor area, and additional scarring.

Correction Albeit tempting, surgical excision of a scar tends to lead to the reappearance of the same scar over time. Placing grafts into the scar can be helpful but sometimes the blood supply is poor and may not be entirely beneficial. Use of micropigmentation (tattooing) can also help cover the previous scarring. Chronic nerve pain (or conversely permanent anesthesia) that can arise from inadvertent transection of occipital nerves can be addressed with targeted botulinum-toxin injections into the specific area of discomfort. After 1 to 2 sessions of neurotoxin (2–5 units), the patient can be afforded lasting relief.

Recipient Site

Complication
Pitting (**Fig. 1**).

Cause The graft was placed too deep relative to the surrounding tissue.

Avoidance The graft should fit the site correctly, and test grafts should always be undertaken first

to ensure that the graft-to-site fit is appropriate before major graft dissection is undertaken. The graft should fit so that it rests approximately 1 mm above the surrounding skin because when the edema resolves, the graft settles to be flush with the surrounding skin. If placed flush or lower than the surrounding skin, the site has a greater likelihood of eventual pitting.

Correction It is very hard to correct pitting. In sensitive areas like the hairline, if the hairline is at the appropriate position or too low, then the grafts can be removed through punch excision. Otherwise, additional grafts can be placed around the bad grafts to camouflage them in an approach known as "de-emphasis grafting."

Complication
Cobblestoning.

Cause Cobblestoning is the opposite problem of pitting. When grafts are placed too high to the surrounding scalp, they can create a cobblestoned appearance (ie, raised vis-à-vis the surrounding scalp).

Avoidance Grafts must be placed that fit the site correctly. If the grafts are too large, they may not settle into the site correctly and thereby leave a cobblestoned appearance after wound healing.

Correction Cobblestoning is very hard to correct. The cobblestoned area can be transected flush to the scalp or more grafts can be used to be placed around the existing bad grafts through "de-emphasis grafting."

Complication
Compression (see **Fig. 1**).

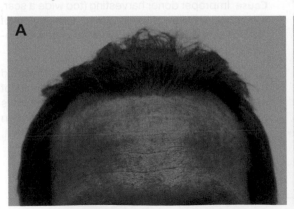
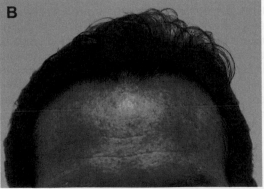

Fig. 1. Multiple aesthetic problems including a hairline that is too round and straight, grafts that are too large and that are placed into the hairline, as well as pitting and compression of the grafts. He is shown after a corrective hair-transplant procedure with a much more natural result. (*A*) The image before corrective work and (*B*) the result after corrective hair transplant.

Cause Grafts with numerous hairs and that are too large for a particular site can be squeezed together to appear as a central tuft of hair, almost like a plug of yesteryear.

Avoidance Ensure that grafts fit the site appropriately.

Correction Similar to the correction stated above in "pitting."

Complication
Kinky hair (**Fig. 2**).

Cause The hair shaft is overly manipulated or crushed during insertion by the grasping forceps leading to a wiry hair growth.

Avoidance The graft should be held only by the surrounding fat cuff and never on the hair shaft itself.

Correction Correction is similar to the correction stated above in "pitting."

Complication
Poor growth (**Fig. 3**).

Avoidance Patients must understand that sometimes, despite a surgeon's best efforts, growth can be underwhelming based on a patient's growth characteristics. However, certain factors can predispose toward poor growth including not using recipient tumescent solution (0.01% lidocaine with 1:500,000 epinephrine) to protect the underlying neurovasculature, implanting grafts into too dense a distribution, and poor handling and manipulation of grafts (as mentioned above in pitting and kinky hair). Use of PRP during a procedure can improve a patient's chance of success with hair growth in the author's experience.

Correction A second hair transplant may need to be performed with better technique.

Complication
Unnatural hairline (see **Figs. 1–3**; **Fig. 4**).

Cause An unnatural hairline can arise from a host of problems that involve a badly positioned hairlinen (too low, too high, improper slope, too wide, too narrow, and does not match a natural Norwood pattern of hair loss), too straight or harsh (use of grafts that are too large in the frontal hairline, not angling the grafts correctly [see **Fig. 4**], not creating a natural micro-undulating hairline, not putting "sentinel" one-hair grafts to soften the hairline), or having any of the problems like pitting, kinky hair, and so on, mentioned above.

Avoidance The macro hairline (the line drawn on the head) should be undertaken only after a surgeon understands the natural Norwood patterns and can construct a hairline based on accepted principles that mimic nature. The micro hairline (the actual recipient sites and grafts placed) must be constructed with utmost care so that the angles are low and straightforward and appear to look like a cragged coastline (ie, without appearing too straight and harsh). The assistants who place grafts must adhere to careful attention to avoid previously enumerated problems, including pitting, kinky hair, placement of inappropriate graft sizes for a particular location, poor growth, and similar problems.

Correction If the hairline is too high, the hairline can be redrawn lower and a better designed and constructed hairline can be placed in front of the bad grafts to camouflage them ("de-emphasis grafting") (see **Figs. 1–3**). If the hairline is too low to be acceptable or natural in appearance, then grafts can be punched out that reside in front of

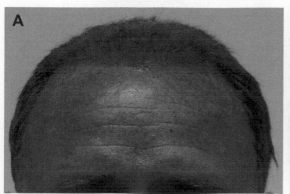
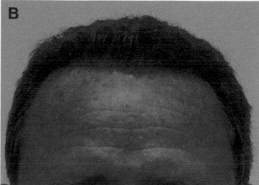

Fig. 2. Hair transplant in which the hairline is too straight and round as well as grafts that are too large placed into the hairline. In addition, the hair appears kinky due to overmanipulation of the hair grafts during insertion. He is shown after a corrective hair transplant result with a much improved, natural result. (*A*) The image before corrective work and (*B*) the result after corrective hair transplant.

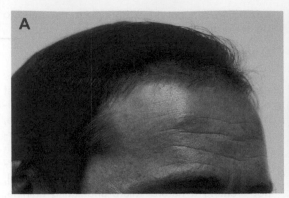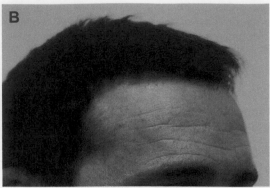

Fig. 3. A hair transplant that showed poor growth, unnatural hair angles (hairs were transplanted in all different directions), and large pluglike grafts (most likely under compression) and was corrected with a hair transplant procedure that shows a more natural result and much greater visual density. (*A*) The image before corrective work and (*B*) the result after corrective hair transplant.

the proposed new hairline. Alternatively, a strip of grafts can be excised from the hairline to raise the hairline upward, after which time when the wound is well healed, a new hairline can be constructed according to the meticulous principles of good hairline design and execution.

Complication
Necrosis/poor scalp healing. Poor scalp healing can manifest as a hypopigmented scalp, a chronically discolored scalp, or frank necrosis.

Cause Besides a patient's predisposing factors, such as smoking, chronic sun damage, and diabetes, a surgeon can inflict this outcome when the underlying vasculature is carelessly transected during recipient-site creation.

Avoidance Use of proper recipient-tumescent fluid is important to increase the distance between

the recipient-site creating instrument (eg, needle, blade) and the underlying neurovasculature. Also, avoiding overdense packing (>50 sites per cm^2) may help to minimize this problem. For signs of venous congestion or incipient necrosis, using nitropaste can be an immeasurably important rescue tactic. As mentioned earlier, use of PRP injected into the scalp an hour or so before site creation can help improve wound-healing capacity and minimize this risk. In patients who are very bald and have signs of poor vascularization, use of topical minoxidil for several months may anecdotally improve blood supply to the target recipient area but no conclusive studies have been undertaken to demonstrate that benefit.

Correction If the scalp looks discolored or hypopigmented in some way, additional grafts (placed in a more careful manner explained above and

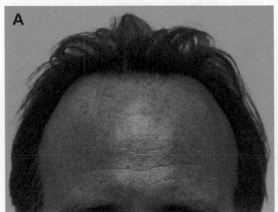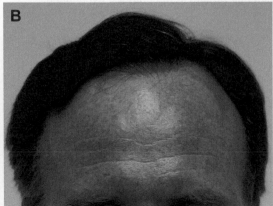

Fig. 4. A hair transplant that lacks density and a hairline that appears natural for 3 reasons: grafts are too large in the hairline; hairline design is too straight and, most obviously, hair angles are placed almost perpendicular to the scalp rather than more appropriately at a low, forward, acute angle. He is shown after a corrective procedure with a much more natural hairline and hair-transplant result. (*A*) The image before corrective work and (*B*) the result after corrective hair transplant.

only undertaken a year or more later to allow for wound healing) may camouflage the scalp appearance. However, clearly the concern is compromising the blood supply further from additional transplantation. Use of minoxidil postoperatively may also help revitalize the scalp. In cases of frank necrosis, the eschar should be left in place (not debrided for fear that the tenuous blood supply is further compromised) and kept moistened with an antibiotic solution. When the eschar sloughs, the surgeon can consider excision of the necrosis or grafting into the area preferably many months to a year later. As an alternative, micropigmentation of the scalp can be performed to camouflage the area of baldness.

PROCEDURAL APPROACH

The complications that arise during hair restoration can be divided between donor site (which is the exclusive responsibility of the surgeon) and the recipient site (which is the result of both surgeon and assistant quality of care), as illustrated in the preceding section. Unlike almost any other cosmetic surgical enterprise, a hair-transplant procedure is highly dependent on the skill of the assistant to generate a result of uncompromising quality. As good surgical outcome is predicated on good surgical technique (for both the surgeon and the assistant), it is paramount to understand that every minute task must be carried out flawlessly. Unfortunately, to describe the elaborate procedural detail that would have any merit for the reader so as to avoid complications would require an entire textbook. As this concise monograph simply cannot accommodate that exhaustive narrative, the goal is to describe in broader strokes the principles behind what causes many of the major potentially avoidable complications that can arise during hair transplantation.

The donor area must be treated with great respect because compromise in this area can lead to permanent numbness, nerve pain, scarring, and a destroyed precious finite donor bank.

Procedural Planning

Careful planning of the donor area to remain within what is known as the "safe zone" (approximately at the occipital protuberance or above but well below the fringe where crown hair loss may encroach) is a prerequisite that requires a surgeon project forward in time what will remain within these confines with ongoing hair loss.

Anesthetic

Use of a tumescent solution (0.01% lidocaine with 1:200,000 epinephrine) typically with about 150 to 250 mL rapidly infused into the subcutaneous planes immediately before harvesting is one of the most important steps in limiting the aforementioned damage to the donor area. The best metaphor to understand how tumescence works is how a ship (the harvesting blade) riding over a coral reef (the underlying neurovasculature) does not harm or scrape the reef at high tide (tumescent solution) but can easily damage the coral at low tide (no tumescent solution).

Hair Harvest

Many surgeons also rush through the process of harvesting the hair from the back of the head, transecting hairs as they go, which can in turn lead to a destruction of many of the hairs, make graft dissection a very arduous task, and lead to poor wound healing. It is imperative that a surgeon evaluate the depth and angle of the harvest so that his blades cause limited hair transection during harvesting. Making micro-adjustments in blade angle and depth in a slow, deliberate fashion can help to avoid much of potential problems in the donor area.

Hairline Design

As previously mentioned, recipient site problems can be divided into surgeon and assistant errors. On the part of the surgeon, it can be further subdivided into problems with hairline design and recipient-site creation. To create an excellent hairline that is natural, fits a patient well, and ages well for that person requires much more sophistication than would be suggested at a cursory glance.

First and foremost, the author always encourages neophyte surgeons to review the Norwood classification for male pattern baldness and to look at individuals who are in various stages of hair recession so that when these new surgeons create a hairline the result will be something that resembles a pattern that exists in nature.

There are 2 levels of mastery:

1. The first step is drawing a hairline that would look natural based on tilt, position, and shape. The hairline must not rest on the vertical plane of the scalp (ie, the forehead but conversely should not be so high as not to frame the face properly), should tilt naturally (from a profile view the hairline should not slope downward from anterior to posterior but either slope upward or stay flat), and should terminate no farther lateral than the lateral canthus from the frontal view.
2. The second level of concern is designing a hairline that truly fits an individual's facial shape,

ethnicity, gender, age, and degree of recession. The author emphasizes this when acolyte surgeons are taught so that they can begin to understand the complexities that exist to create superior hairline design.

As far as recipient-site errors are concerned, the surgeon again must truly understand how hair naturally grows across the scalp of the head. One of the most common errors seen in hairline design is that the angles are placed too high (perpendicular) vis-à-vis the anterior scalp (see **Fig. 4**), which can limit visual density and also reveal the grafts as grafts because one can easily detect the insertion point into the scalp. Recipient-site creation of the hairline also mandates a high level of skill and artistry. The image of a coastline that looks relatively straight when seen from a distant aerial shot but becomes ever more rugged and irregular on closer inspection is a fair comparison. This irregular design that is not readily apparent from a distance but obvious close-up is a way to describe how to effectively make recipient sites along the hairline.

Surgical Technicians

The surgical assistants, or technicians, who help a surgeon in the task of hair restoration are principally delegated to perform 2 major duties:

1. Graft dissection, which involves dividing the donor strip first into single row slivers (like cutting a loaf of bread into slices) and then into individual grafts. Quality grafts that are a product of graft dissection are a prerequisite for an excellent hair-transplant outcome. If grafts are poorly dissected (hairs transected, grafts overly manipulated during dissection, overly trimmed, under trimmed), the grafts can grow out poorly or not at all.

2. Graft placement, which is also a very demanding skill that must be mastered over many months to years on the part of the assistant team. Poor graft placement can lead to poor growth or very unnatural results like pitting (see **Fig. 1**) and kinky hair growth (see **Fig. 2**). The principles of good graft placement involve ensuring proper graft-to-site fit, minimal manipulation, the right-sized graft that fits the right-sized site, and the curl of the hair facing the right direction. The hair curl refers to the natural curvature of the hair shaft as it exits the scalp. The curl should be facing downward and forward when inserted, otherwise the result is that hair that is more difficult to comb or appears unnatural.

SUMMARY

Quality hair restoration requires an understanding and adherence to good technique for both the surgeon and the assistant. Treating hair restoration as a serious surgical endeavor and working hard to attain mastery at this skill through each successive year in practice can lead to improved patient outcomes.

FURTHER READING

Lam SM, Karamanovski E. Hair transplant 360. Delhi (India): Jaypee Brothers; 2011.

Index

Note: Page numbers of article titles are in **boldface** type.

Facial Plast Surg Clin N Am 21 (2013) 681–693
http://dx.doi.org/10.1016/S1064-7406(13)00151-X
1064-7406/13/$ – see front matter © 2013 Elsevier Inc. All rights reserved.

United States Postal Service

Statement of Ownership, Management, and Circulation
(All Periodicals Publications Except Requester Publications)

1. Publication Title	2. Publication Number	3. Filing Date
Facial Plastic Surgery Clinics of North America	0 1 3 - 1 2 2	9/14/13

4. Issue Frequency	5. Number of Issues Published Annually	6. Annual Subscription Price
Feb, May, Aug, Nov	4	$373.00

7. Complete Mailing Address of Known Office of Publication (Not printer) (Street, city, county, state, and ZIP+4®)

Elsevier Inc.
360 Park Avenue South
New York, NY 10010-1710

Contact Person
Stephen Bushing
Telephone (Include area code)
215-239-3688

8. Complete Mailing Address of Headquarters or General Business Office of Publisher (Not printer)

Elsevier Inc., 360 Park Avenue South, New York, NY 10010-1710

9. Full Names and Complete Mailing Addresses of Publisher, Editor, and Managing Editor (Do not leave blank)

Publisher (Name and complete mailing address)

Linda Belfus, Elsevier, Inc., 1600 John F. Kennedy Blvd. Suite 1800, Philadelphia, PA 19103-2899

Editor (Name and complete mailing address)

Joanne Husovski, Elsevier, Inc., 1600 John F. Kennedy Blvd. Suite 1800, Philadelphia, PA 19103-2899

Managing Editor (Name and complete mailing address)

Barbara Cohen - Kligerman, Elsevier, Inc., 1600 John F. Kennedy Blvd. Suite 1800, Philadelphia, PA 19103-2899

10. Owner (Do not leave blank. If the publication is owned by a corporation, give the name and address of the corporation immediately followed by the names and addresses of all stockholders owning or holding 1 percent or more of the total amount of stock. If not owned by a corporation, give the names and addresses of the individual owners. If owned by a partnership or other unincorporated firm, give its name and address as well as those of each individual owner. If the publication is published by a nonprofit organization, give its name and address.)

Full Name	Complete Mailing Address
Wholly owned subsidiary of	1600 John F. Kennedy Blvd., Ste. 1800
Reed/Elsevier, US holdings	Philadelphia, PA 19103-2899

11. Known Bondholders, Mortgagees, and Other Security Holders Owning or Holding 1 Percent or More of Total Amount of Bonds, Mortgages, or Other Securities. If none, check box.   ☐ None

Full Name	Complete Mailing Address
N/A	

12. Tax Status (For completion by nonprofit organizations authorized to mail at nonprofit rates) (Check one)
The purpose, function, and nonprofit status of this organization and the exempt status for federal income tax purposes:
☐ Has Not Changed During Preceding 12 Months
☐ Has Changed During Preceding 12 Months (Publisher must submit explanation of change with this statement)

PS Form 3526, September 2007 (Page 1 of 3 (Instructions Page 3))   PSN 7530-01-000-9931 PRIVACY NOTICE: See our Privacy policy in www.usps.com

---

13. Publication Title	14. Issue Date for Circulation Data Below
Facial Plastic Surgery Clinics of North America	May 2013

15. Extent and Nature of Circulation		Average No. Copies Each Issue During Preceding 12 Months	No. Copies of Single Issue Published Nearest to Filing Date
a. Total Number of Copies (Net press run)		569	493
b. Paid Circulation (By Mail and Outside the Mail)	(1) Mailed Outside-County Paid Subscriptions Stated on PS Form 3541. (Include paid distribution above nominal rate, advertiser's proof copies, and exchange copies)	297	275
	(2) Mailed In-County Paid Subscriptions Stated on PS Form 3541 (Include paid distribution above nominal rate, advertiser's proof copies, and exchange copies)		
	(3) Paid Distribution Outside the Mails Including Sales Through Dealers and Carriers, Street Vendors, Counter Sales, and Other Paid Distribution Outside USPS®	61	48
	(4) Paid Distribution by Other Classes Mailed Through the USPS (e.g. First-Class Mail®)		
c. Total Paid Distribution (Sum of 15b (1), (2), (3), and (4))	▲	358	279
d. Free or Nominal Rate Distribution (By Mail and Outside the Mail)	(1) Free or Nominal Rate Outside-County Copies Included on PS Form 3541	78	50
	(2) Free or Nominal Rate In-County Copies Included on PS Form 3541		
	(3) Free or Nominal Rate Copies Mailed at Other Classes Through the USPS (e.g. First-Class Mail)		
	(4) Free or Nominal Rate Distribution Outside the Mail (Carriers or other means)		
e. Total Free or Nominal Rate Distribution (Sum of 15d (1), (2), (3) and (4))	▲	78	50
f. Total Distribution (Sum of 15c and 15e)	▲	436	329
g. Copies not Distributed (See instructions to publishers #4 (page #3))	▲	133	164
h. Total (Sum of 15f and g)		569	493
i. Percent Paid (15c divided by 15f times 100)		82.11%	84.80%

16. Publication of Statement of Ownership

☐ If the publication is a general publication, publication of this statement is required. Will be printed in the November 2013 issue of this publication.   ☐ Publication not required

17. Signature and Title of Editor, Publisher, Business Manager, or Owner	Date
[signature] Stephen R. Bushing –Inventory/Distribution Coordinator	September 14, 2013

I certify that all information furnished on this form is true and complete. I understand that anyone who furnishes false or misleading information on this form or who omits material or information requested on the form may be subject to criminal sanctions (including fines and imprisonment) and/or civil sanctions (including civil penalties).

PS Form 3526, September 2007 (Page 2 of 3)

Printed and bound by CPI Group (UK) Ltd, Croydon, CR0 4YY

03/10/2024

01040309-0012